Praise for
The Planet Friendly Diet

The Planet Friendly Diet is the new "diet bible" and it complements everyone's daily routine in diet and exercise. With a bright, fresh perspective and well-rounded view on health and how to maintain it, it's the book I travel around the world with!

— Kylie Bax, supermodel and Mum

The Planet Friendly Diet has many benefits, including reducing exposure to pesticides and toxins found in animal fats and processed foods. This reduction — together with the beneficial effects for your body's detoxification pathways of many of the vegetables, fruits, and spices in the food plan — helps reduce your body's toxic load.

— Dr. Karen van Wyk, MD

The Planet Friendly Diet is an excellent introduction to improving your body composition, and the quality of your diet. ... I encourage you to look after yourself by putting this book into practice.

— Dr. Chris Smiley, MD

I feel so lucky to have come to Whistler and experienced *The Planet Friendly Diet*. It made me realize that I can do dinner in just 15 minutes! Very easy to cook and the portions are huge. I've been eating meat for breakfast, lunch, and dinner my whole life, and I didn't know if I could *not* eat meat, but then I did it, and I feel so much better.

— Gloria Chen, Taiwan

You'll end up making many of the recipes over and over again — simple healthy recipes to make. If you want to be healthy, stay fit, lose weight, get rid of bad food choices, *The Planet Friendly Diet* is your book — go ahead and give it a try. You won't be disappoint

a)

D1275731

10

Highly recommended for the serious d wishes to enhance an already healthful re

— Wanda Urbanska, simplicity advocate and co-author, *Less is More*

We all know "we are what we eat," but less often considered is the fact the Earth reflects our diet choices as well — and it's in poor shape. *The Planet Friendly Diet* connects the dots between a healthy environment and a healthy body. If more of us read this book and followed its sensible and inspiring message to eat as if the world depended on it, we'd all be better off.

— David Tracey, author, *Urban Agriculture*

The Planet Friendly Diet is truly a lifestyle. ...this book has shown me how to combine foods and how to prepare them in healthy ways. I really like how it explains the macronutrients in real-life terms so you can bring it into your own diet. I feel like I can help my children and friends to eat healthier; the knowledge I've gained is something that I will share with everybody.

— Kathy Lovett, Yellow Knife (Canada)

Powerful, practical, and personal, this book brings the inspiring and authentic Cat Smiley into your own kitchen as mentor and motivator. Do good for your body and the planet, and feel the change after just 21 days? That's the plan we need to kick-start a healthy change in our world.

— Lisa Kivirist, author, *Soil Sisters: A Toolkit for Women Farmers* and
*Homemade for Sale: How to Set Up and
Market a Food Business from Your Home Kitchen*

This is a must-read for anyone seeking a realistic alternative to fad diets or cold-turkey transitions into weight loss or health overhauls.

— Nicole Caldwell, CEO, Better Farm, and author,
Better: The Everyday Art of Sustainable Living

I've been on *The Planet Friendly Diet* now for five weeks and have lost 40 pounds — wahoo! The food is delicious, the smoothies especially. You've got to try it to believe it. It's been a life altering experience, and normally I would be a little nervous about finishing a diet and continuing but with this amazing book I know that I will continue to stay on track. Thanks Cat!

— Hardeep Atwal, Vancouver, Canada

the planet friendly diet

YOUR 21-DAY GUIDE TO sustainable weight loss and optimal health

CAT SMILEY

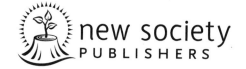

new society
PUBLISHERS

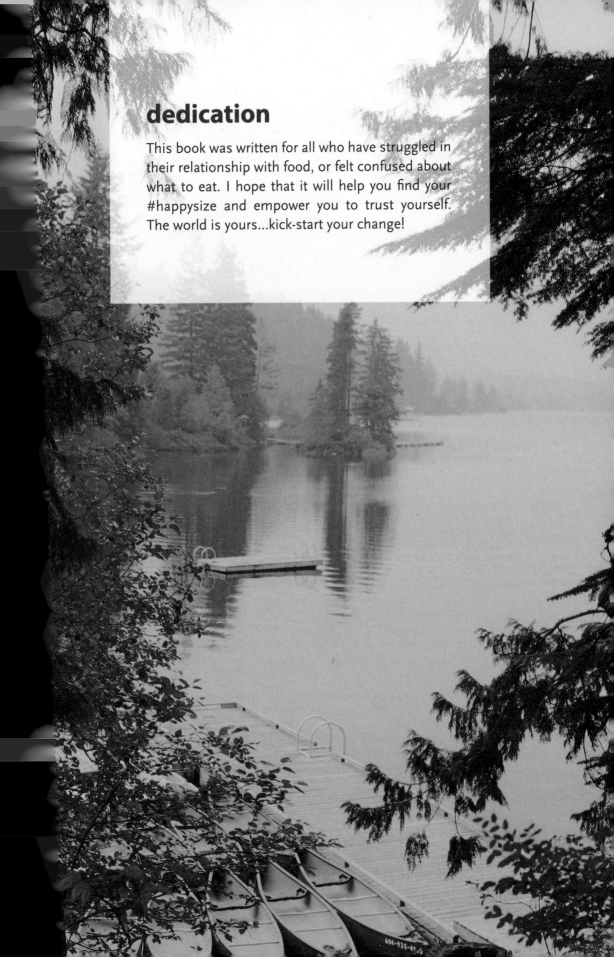

dedication

This book was written for all who have struggled in their relationship with food, or felt confused about what to eat. I hope that it will help you find your #happysize and empower you to trust yourself. The world is yours...kick-start your change!

Cover design by Emma Moldrich adapted by Diane McIntosh.

Interior design by Emma Moldrich adapted by MJ Jessen. Photographs courtesy of Cat Smiley, Darby Magill, Chris Smiley, Aimee and Thomas Smiley, Louis Charles. Food styling and recipe creation by Cat Smiley. Stock images courtesy of www.sxc.hu. Social media icons © Zee Que | Designbolts.com. Cork Board — AdobeStock_92101856

Printed in Canada. First printing January 2016
2014 edition © Cat Smiley Unlimited. All rights reserved.

Funded by the Government of Canada   Financé par le gouvernement du Canada | **Canada**

This book is intended to be educational and informative. The author and publisher disclaim all responsibility for any liability, loss or risk that may be associated with the application of any of the contents of this book, personal or otherwise, which may occur from taking action on any content contained in this book. This publication contains the opinions and ideas of the author and is not intended to replace the advice of medical professionals.

Paperback ISBN: 978-0-86571-811-1
eISBN: 978-1-55092-608-8

Inquiries regarding requests to reprint all or part of *The Planet Friendly Diet* should be addressed to New Society Publishers at the address below. To order directly from the publishers, please call toll-free (North America) 1-800-567-6772, or order online at www.newsociety.com

Any other inquiries can be directed by mail to:
New Society Publishers
P.O. Box 189, Gabriola Island, BC V0R 1X0, Canada
(250) 247-9737

New Society Publishers' mission is to publish books that contribute in fundamental ways to building an ecologically sustainable and just society, and to do so with the least possible impact on the environment, in a manner that models this vision. We are committed to doing this not just through education, but through action. The interior pages of our bound books are printed on Forest Stewardship Council®-registered acid-free paper that is **100% post-consumer recycled** (100% old growth forest-free), processed chlorine-free, and printed with vegetable-based, low-VOC inks, with covers produced using FSC®-registered stock. New Society also works to reduce its carbon footprint, and purchases carbon offsets based on an annual audit to ensure a carbon neutral footprint. For further information, or to browse our full list of books and purchase securely, visit our website at: www.newsociety.com

Library and Archives Canada Cataloguing in Publication

Smiley, Cat, author
    The planet friendly diet : your 21-day guide to sustainable weight loss and optimal health / Cat Smiley.

Originally published: Createspace, 2011.
Includes bibliographical references and index. Issued in print and electronic formats.
ISBN 978-0-86571-811-1 (paperback).--ISBN 978-1-55092-608-8 (ebook)

    1. Reducing diets--Recipes. 2. Cooking (Natural foods). 3. Sustainable living.
4. Nutrition. 5. Cookbooks. I. Title.

RM222.2.S534 2016   641.5'63   C2015-904660-2
                                           C2015-904661-0

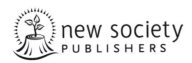

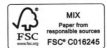

new society PUBLISHERS

FSC   MIX   Paper from responsible sources   www.fsc.org   FSC® C016245

contents

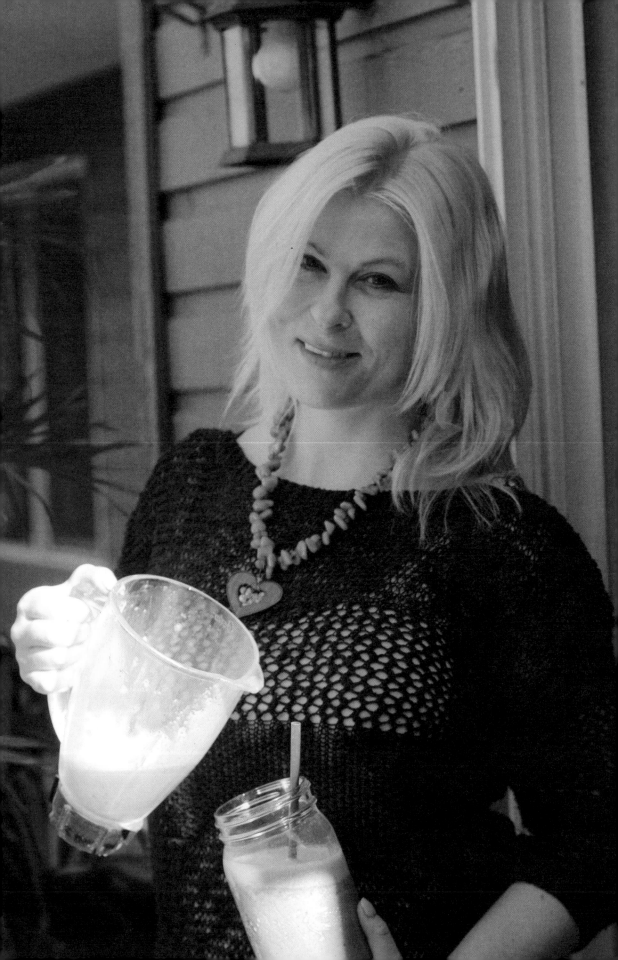

introduction

The Planet Friendly Diet was born back in 2008, when I moved my boot camp business into a weight-loss retreat (*Whistler Fitness Vacations*). Women were joining our live-in program for 1–12 weeks to focus full time on losing weight and getting fit — with food an integral part of it, I needed fresh learning material for the nutrition seminars. These guests were up to 200 pounds overweight, often addicted to sugar and processed foods. Quite different from the super healthy boot camp clientele I'd worked with for the past ten years! I wanted to introduce them to our West Coast kale and chia-seed world, moving away from the government's food pyramid/rainbow. It was met with a constant fight. I had to do better.... I had to think of a way to sell them on the idea of sustainable nutrition, without making them think that their meat-and-potato diet was wrong. As I started writing out my reasons, the words kept getting more and more confusing. I realized in order to re-educate, I needed to start from the beginning. But what was the beginning? How on earth was I going to break down such a huge topic? It felt like an overwhelming task — but I knew it had to be done.

Then one rainy Sunday afternoon while marking food journals for my boot camp clients, I had a lightbulb moment (between 2008 and 2012 I juggled both businesses — boot camp at the crack of dawn, then the weight-loss retreat after that). Here I had in front of me 30 food journals from healthy women who took wheatgrass shots and drank kombucha, baked chia-seed muffins and knew how to cook with almond milk. They were a shining example of what a healthy lifestyle can do for you.

With my boot campers' permission, I put together a small team, including data analysts and dietician students, to review these dietary patterns under a microscope. The study lasted about 2 years. Questions we tried to answer included things like: what macronutrient is dominant at 9am for post-workout snack if their 6am breakfast was oatmeal and blueberries? We found consistency in almost 500 exercisers of healthy weight that protein cravings kicked in when it was missing from the meal eaten prior. When we asked the same people to switch to quinoa oats and use soy instead of almond milk, for example, although the calorie count was increased, so was the protein, which resulted in them usually opting for fruit at 9am instead of their previous higher-energy snack. There were dozens of case studies like these that we looked at, in an effort to come up with the **new "food rules"**.

We got to a point in the study where we saw wheatgrass shots and sprouted grain toast in scientific numbers. These were transferred into ridiculous amounts of Excel sheets, translated into layman's terms, discussed at roundtables and formulated into conclusions. The sustainable modern diet had now officially been dissected, and the results were nothing short of spectacular. It was like discovering a gold mine. While there were a ton of books out there on "how to go vegan" etc., there didn't seem to be many "how to eat" books on nutrition science and how it relates to sustainable food choices for gluten-, wheat-, dairy- and soy-free plant-based diets. It was a book I needed to write.

Fast-forward to today, I'd love to tell this story with an upbeat middle part where I skipped off into a publishing deal with my great big awesome idea and everything worked out. Alas, despite my booming business and people flying in from all over the world to work with me, this constant environment of guiding people in their food choices sunk me on a downward spiral in my own. Since the age of 14, I had struggled with exercise addiction, body image issues and disordered eating, around the same time I quit meat cold turkey. The concept of eating animals had always made me really upset! Although I went on to become an "acclaimed body transformation coach" and top athlete, it was easy to take care of everyone else's struggles instead of dealing with my own. Perhaps I was vicariously recovering through them, I don't know, but as I slimmed them down to skinnier than my perceived goal weight and high-fived their victories, I started to ask myself...*why do I feel stuck?*

Then something remarkable happened.

The first few seasons, *Whistler Fitness Vacations* was closed for winter so I seized the opportunity to rekindle my love of traveling and **started to count my blessings over breakfast instead of calories**. Between celebrating my birthday with tsunami orphans in Sri Lanka and feeding street dogs in the slums of Mexico, *The Planet Friendly Diet* book project became my corner of change and recovery happened naturally. I could feel myself becoming a better person, and I liked her! I stopped detoxing, working out like a maniac and being embarrassed about wearing size 12 jeans. Having the opportunity to do small acts of compassion every day (that were unrelated to health and fitness) moved my self-worth away from what I weighed; instead I valued myself based on what I contributed to the world. I realized my voice as an educator could not only take weight off my customers, but also provide a platform that might help them evolve and reconnect with humanity. I figured that the "do-good" factor of eating more compassionately, ethically and more eco-consciously might elevate my clients' sense of self, and kindness would follow towards the way they treated both themselves and the people around them. It could change the world!

I love to think big, and the thought of indirectly saving hundreds of animals from the dinner table just by getting everyone at *Whistler Fitness Vacations* to detox from eating things with a face for a couple of weeks was definately an idea worth sharing. Suddenly my book had a soul, and I realized how important it was for me.

It was such an exciting time getting the project to where it is now. My blog catsmiley.com became the hub of the books progress, as I taught myself how to become a better vegetarian chef, food stylist and photographer. As my readership grew, so did my motivation. Eating was fun again — the plate in front of me became a work of art, instead of being the enemy! I thought that sharing my ideas on nutrition might help others heal, but never did I expect it to help *me* heal. What a great lesson.

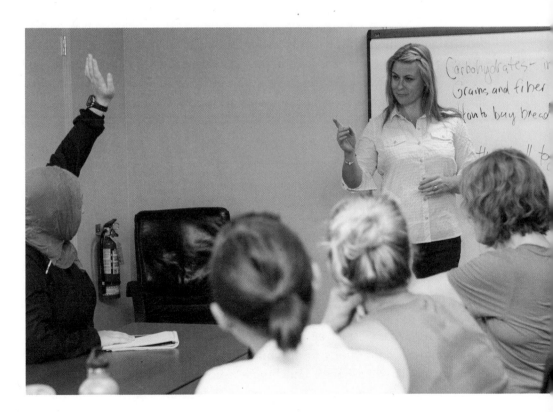

This introduction wouldn't be complete without expressing my gratitude to those who made it possible. There were so many people who played a part — wonderful clients who went through my recipes with red marker circling typos, adding spice suggestions, marking errors and feedback. This was so encouraging! To my publishers, New Society, who saw the potential in this book and helped bring it to more homes worldwide. To those on my Facebook page who voted on image selections, recipe names — and cheered for me when I got a book deal. Thank you as well to those who contributed success stories and testimonials, plus told your daughters and mothers about the principles in this book. It's super-cool to have had a small influence on your food choices.

I'm eternally grateful also to my wonderful parents for raising me on wholesome food and teaching me about healthy lifestyle from a young age. Also for being fearless travelers which most definitely inspired my path! And most importantly of all, along this journey of countless editions, late nights and rewrites, my incredible man Louis was there celebrating the progress, pep-talking me, giving my life balance and making me laugh until our fur-child Manchas looked like he was laughing too. Those guys are seriously the most "crazy love of my not-so-normal world" — my everything.

It's been a family project on both a professional and personal level, and it is a great honor for me that you are holding this book in your hands. I hope that *The Planet Friendly Diet* will ignite your fire to take better care of yourself, try new adventures, love your body and be the person you want to be. Enjoy the journey and embrace your #happysize! I wish you luck.

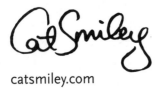

catsmiley.com

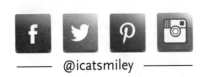

—— @icatsmiley ——

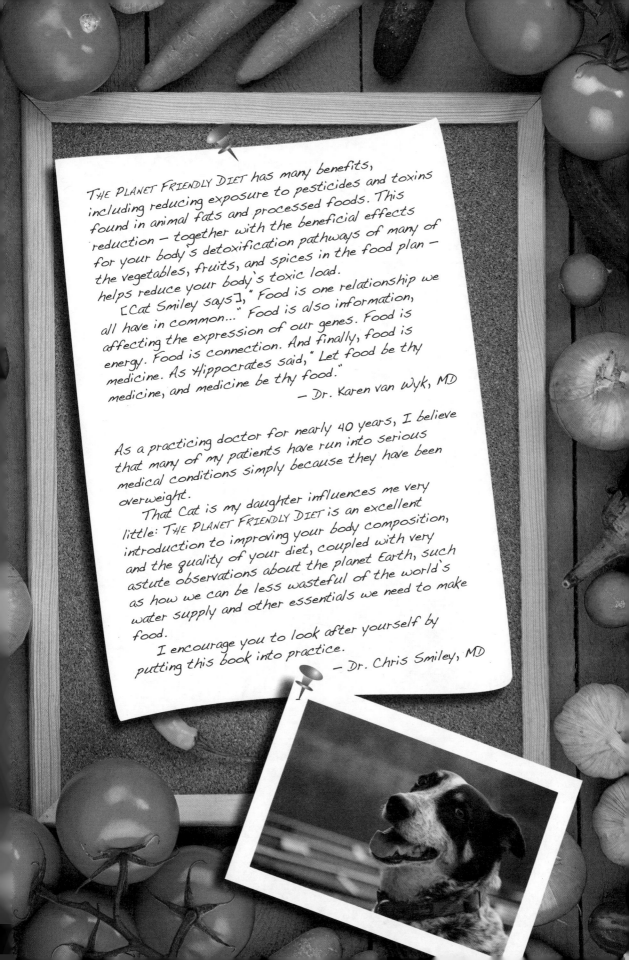

THE PLANET FRIENDLY DIET has many benefits, including reducing exposure to pesticides and toxins found in animal fats and processed foods. This reduction — together with the beneficial effects for your body's detoxification pathways of many of the vegetables, fruits, and spices in the food plan — helps reduce your body's toxic load.

[Cat Smiley says], "Food is one relationship we all have in common..." Food is also information, affecting the expression of our genes. Food is energy. Food is connection. And finally, food is medicine. As Hippocrates said, "Let food be thy medicine, and medicine be thy food."

— Dr. Karen van Wyk, MD

As a practicing doctor for nearly 40 years, I believe that many of my patients have run into serious medical conditions simply because they have been overweight.

That Cat is my daughter influences me very little: THE PLANET FRIENDLY DIET is an excellent introduction to improving your body composition, and the quality of your diet, coupled with very astute observations about the planet Earth, such as how we can be less wasteful of the world's water supply and other essentials we need to make food.

I encourage you to look after yourself by putting this book into practice.

— Dr. Chris Smiley, MD

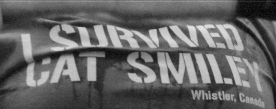

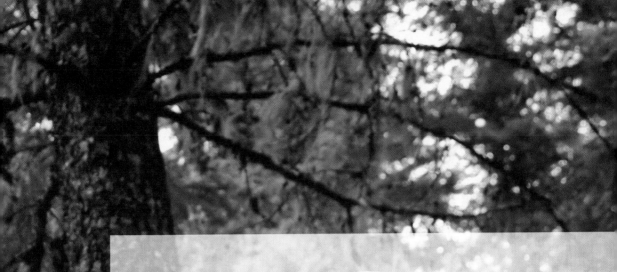

week 1

My nutrition philosophy is about getting back to basics with the natural foods of the soil. I target natural weight loss through increased fruits and vegetables, providing all the nutrition, vitamins, minerals, fiber, fats, proteins and carbohydrates needed to lose weight and keep it off — without starving yourself. The goal is to increase nutrient assimilation by blending specific produce together to break down the cells of plants and improve digestibility by unlocking the raw nutrients.

The Planet Friendly Diet includes two smoothies per day and one meal — 1,200 healthy calories per day that are high in phytonutrients and antioxidants. You'll experience mental clarity and focus, in addition to increased energy, weight loss, clearer skin and reduced cravings for unhealthy foods. We focus on alkaline foods that will rebalance your body and maintain pH levels, while including chlorophyll-rich foods every day, which will help purify your blood and boost your immune system. You'll become an expert on nutrition science with the comprehensive lessons in this book that will empower your eating choices and help you make your own healthy dietary decisions.

Kick-start your change by eating clean for at least 7 days prior to starting *The Planet Friendly Diet*. You may wish to complete a cleanse if coming from a background of toxins — stress, junk food, sugar, salt, fat, excessive caffeine, cigarettes, pollution, alcohol. Starting your program with a clean slate will maximize the benefits. If you're not doing a cleanse prior to starting the program, minimize consumption of breads, flour, sugar, dairy, alcohol, caffeine and fermented foods like soy sauce, wine and miso soup. Use this experience to open your mind and inner connection.

Ready to get started? Read these next couple of pages first — there are important tips and details on how to make the staple foods in this plan. Then jump into your Sunday shopping list on page 29 and get started!

tip № 1

get your kitchen ready for cooking

It sounds logical, but if you've been microwaving TV dinners and heating up takeout in your kitchen, you'll probably need to stock up on the kitchen essentials. Ask friends if they have extra before buying — it might inspire them to de-clutter and organize their kitchen.

- Large stainless steel pan — save calories by reducing the need for oils.
- Large deep pot — for boiling beans and other vegetables.
- Kitchen blender — get a metal-based, glass blender with at least 8 speed settings. It will cost you more, but blenders are not where you want to save money. You'll be making smoothies every day, and a good blender will save sticky explosions and uncrushed strawberries!
- Wooden chopping board — about the size of the sink. I love the big bamboo kinds, or stop by your local farmers' market for one made of native wood.
- Heavy sharp knife — don't buy a cheap one from the grocery store; it'll just cause you frustration. Choose a good one so that you will get into the habit of correct chopping technique and precision right from the beginning of your newfound love of cooking!
- Wooden spoon — anything else will scratch your pan. You're fine to go cheap on this at the grocery store; it's nothing special.
- Airtight containers — for storing leftover portions and food prepared in advance. Buy a bunch, the more the merrier.
- Freezer bags, plastic cling wrap and lots of ice cube trays.
- Aluminum foil — you'll need this for baking fish in the oven to save scrubbing the tray afterwards.

tip no 2

learn to cut fruit and veggies

Wash produce first. Use a good sharp knife to help maintain correct chopping technique and precision. The blade should be at least 1½ inches at the widest point, making it easier to rock the knife on the cutting board while chopping. It's much easier with a big cutting board, about the size of the kitchen sink.

For safety, keep the fruit or vegetable on the cutting board when you chop. Cut down with the knife, while the other hand firmly holds the produce in place. The knuckles should be the closest thing to the knife; curl fingers inwards towards your palm and cut slowly until you gain confidence if you are just starting out.

tip no 3

be food safe

This is such an important part of your planet friendly lifestyle! Learn and memorize all of the guidelines below before venturing into the kitchen. It'll save you some nasty days of foodborne illness and feeling sick. Not what you need when you're trying to do everything right!

Wash hands with warm soapy water for at least 20 seconds before and after handling food, using the washroom and changing diapers. Wash countertops with warm soapy water after preparing each food item. Wash fresh fruits and vegetables under cool drinkable water before eating or cooking them. Use a vegetable scrub brush on produce that has a firm skin, such as carrots, potatoes, melons and squash.

Cut and prepare raw meat, fish and poultry on a separate cutting board from that used to cut vegetables, fruit or other foods. Consider using paper towels to clean up kitchen surfaces. If you use cloth towels, wash often in the hot cycle of your washing machine. For added protection, use a bleach solution to sanitize. Mix 5 mL (1 tsp) of household bleach to 750 mL (3 cups) of water in a labelled spray bottle.

Always place cooked food on a clean plate. Don't use the same plates for raw and cooked meat, poultry, fish or seafood because cross-contamination can occur. Never leave raw meat, poultry, fish, seafood or leftovers out on the counter for longer than two hours. Food that has been defrosted in the microwave should be cooked right away after thawing. Bring gravies, soups and sauces to a full rolling boil and stir during the process.

Wash reusable grocery bags frequently, especially if carrying raw meat, poultry, fish or seafood. If you've used utensils to handle raw food, don't use them again until you've cleaned them thoroughly in the dishwasher or in warm soapy water.

Always remember to cook raw meat, poultry and seafood to a safe internal temperature. Remove from the heat and insert a digital food thermometer through the thickest part of the meat, all the way to the middle and not touching any bones. Avoid consuming any raw or lightly cooked eggs or egg products such as cookie dough or cake batter. Place raw meat, poultry, fish and seafood on the bottom shelf of your refrigerator so raw juices won't drip onto other food. You can cool leftovers quickly by placing them in shallow containers. Refrigerate as soon as possible or within two hours.

Make sure your fridge is set to 4°C (40°F) or lower, and freezer is at −18°C (0°F) or lower. This will keep food out of the temperature danger zone, between 4°C (40°F) and 60°C (140°F), where bacteria can grow quickly. Store cut fruits and vegetables in the fridge.

Defrost raw meat, poultry, fish or seafood in the refrigerator, in a microwave or immersed in cold water. Don't refreeze thawed food! Always store eggs in original carton. Don't pack your fridge with food — cold air must circulate to keep food safe. Check the temperature in your fridge using a thermometer.

Marinate meat in the fridge, not the counter. Don't use leftover marinade from raw food on cooked food. Use a different plate and utensils for raw and cooked meat, poultry, fish or seafood to avoid cross-contamination.

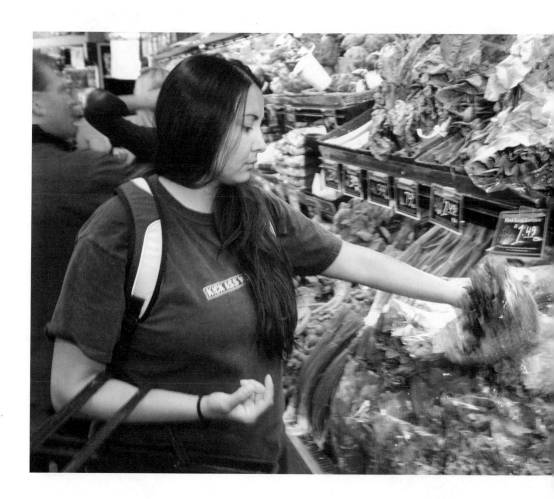

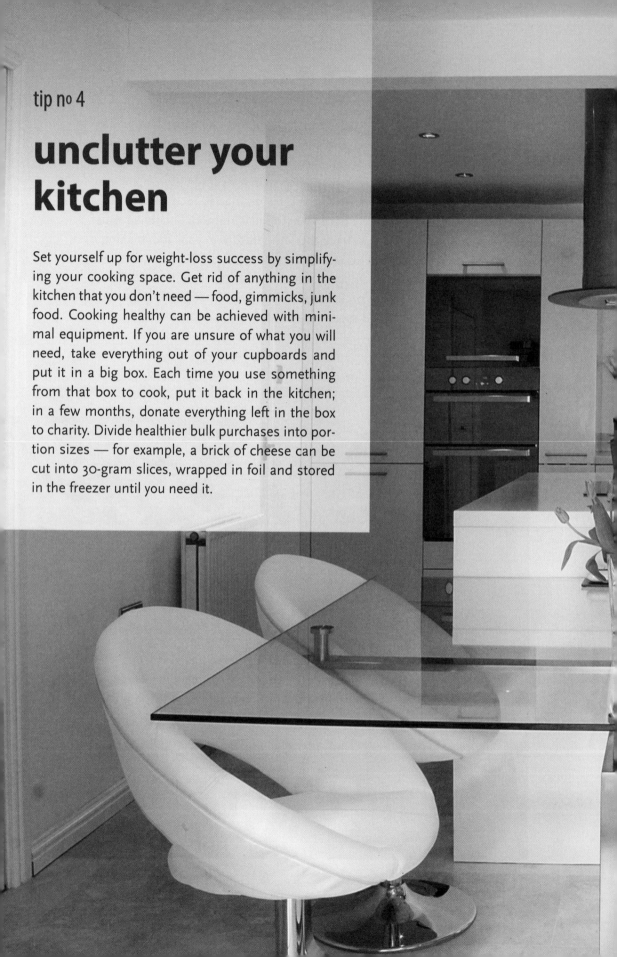

tip nº 4

unclutter your kitchen

Set yourself up for weight-loss success by simplifying your cooking space. Get rid of anything in the kitchen that you don't need — food, gimmicks, junk food. Cooking healthy can be achieved with minimal equipment. If you are unsure of what you will need, take everything out of your cupboards and put it in a big box. Each time you use something from that box to cook, put it back in the kitchen; in a few months, donate everything left in the box to charity. Divide healthier bulk purchases into portion sizes — for example, a brick of cheese can be cut into 30-gram slices, wrapped in foil and stored in the freezer until you need it.

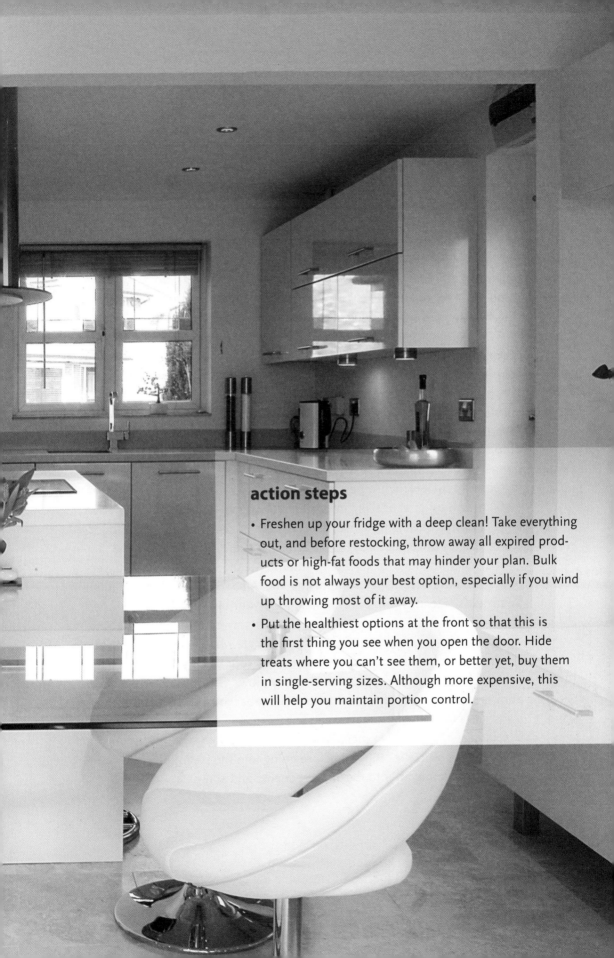

action steps

- Freshen up your fridge with a deep clean! Take everything out, and before restocking, throw away all expired products or high-fat foods that may hinder your plan. Bulk food is not always your best option, especially if you wind up throwing most of it away.

- Put the healthiest options at the front so that this is the first thing you see when you open the door. Hide treats where you can't see them, or better yet, buy them in single-serving sizes. Although more expensive, this will help you maintain portion control.

tip no 5

detox your skin

There's little logic in going meat-free in your diet if you're going to put meat-based products on your skin (like gelatin, an ingredient extracted from animal skin and bone). Skin care is worth the investment, especially during your purification, as it helps your skin function at its best and stay firm while you lose lots of weight. Feeding your skin with botanical pure products is just as important as feeding your appetite with pure food.

Consider using this time of healthy eating to revamp your beauty routine with vegetable-based skin care products. Use products that are reviewed and safety tested for toxic formulas. Vegan-certified products are best because they are never tested on animals and don't contain parabens, gluten and GMO in their formulas.

At *Whistler Fitness Vacations*, many guests use *Arbonne*'s Body Firming Cream and the Awaken Sea Salt Scrub every day with great results. These products (available from catsmiley.com) boost microcirculation, which brings and releases toxins from the skin, exfoliating and stimulating to increase elasticity and firmness while reducing cellulite.

Skin firming is especially important for weight-loss clients who have large amounts of weight to lose, as it will minimize the need for skin-tightening surgery once goal weight has achieved.

It's recommended to take a 10-minute steam, cold shower and second 10-minute steam before applying the *Arbonne* scrubs and cellulite treatments. Steam rooms are amazing for your skin — the pores open up and make it easier for you to sweat and stay cool in your workouts, while enabling your body to effortlessly eliminate whatever toxins that your skin might be holding onto. The heat makes your veins get bigger, which boosts blood flow, giving you that "healthy glow." Steams accelerate stubborn fat loss by emulsifying the fat in your sebaceous glands. You'll know if you carry fat there if you have acne — steams will be especially beneficial in this case. Steams also increase metabolism. Make sure you're on top of your water intake for the day before going into the steam room — drink before, during and after to maximize benefits and stay safe.

tip no 6

set a nutrition schedule

The best way to follow this plan is to set a schedule that works for you. Sticking to the same plan that we do at *Whistler Fitness Vacations* may be an unrealistic goal, but you can modify it to work with your schedule.

Bedtime is early so that guests can be fully energized for the following day; they usually sleep 8 hours or more every night. It's also important that there is 12 hours between dinner and breakfast, so that they can complete their full metabolic cycle.

Upon rising, they weigh first thing after going to the bathroom around 7 am and start drinking their first liter of water while making breakfast (either a smoothie or cooked quinoa oats with blueberries and non-dairy

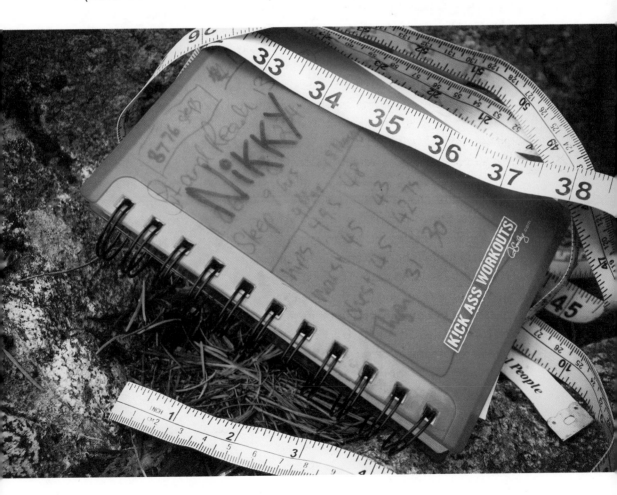

milk). They squeeze fresh lemon into their water and have a cup of black coffee after their smoothie. By about 8:30 am, they've hopefully had a bowel movement, which means that excess waste products are successfully being eliminated and they are ready to start their day of workouts. Bowel movement is really important.

You'll feel much cleaner and energized if you go through this 90-minute routine in the morning, plus it gives you the opportunity to ease into your day gently. Once you start being able to eliminate toxins in the morning, your skin will become clearer.

Between 9 and noon, guests drink their second liter of water, then have 2 more liters before 5 pm. The lunchtime smoothie is 3 hours after breakfast, afternoon snack is 3 hours after lunch, and it's around that time that they have their final bowel movement of the day. Sometimes soup replaces the lunchtime smoothie.

At 5 pm they start cooking dinner and drink a digestive herbal tea in the evening before bed, such as pu'erh, ginger and ginseng organic blend. Go to your local tea store and splurge on your favorite blend!

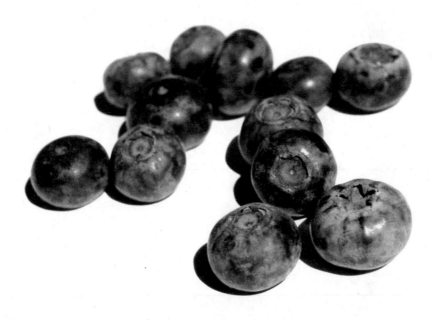

tip nº 7

get medical clearance to start exercising

If you are 30 lb. or more overweight, before doing anything book a medical evaluation to get clearance. They will check both your heart rate and blood pressure to determine the state of your cardiovascular system, and if exercise will place you at risk, plus family history. These are key indicators as to your ability to start exercise and your initial intensity.

Ease into exercise gradually — we can't stress this enough. By preparing gradually through gentle walking and swimming, you'll achieve anatomical adaptation: a process that prepares connective tissues (ligaments and tendons) for the increased tension that shaping up will place on them. Strengthening your connective tissues will decrease the risk of injury and prepare you for unrestricted training and maximum results once you are physically ready.

It's highly recommended to book a few sessions with a personal trainer to guide you in the right direction in the beginning and to keep you motivated for the first couple of weeks while you build up strength.

If you're a parent, shaping up will have huge impact on the way your kids view their own health, helping them live free of heart disease, obesity, diabetes and other obesity-related diseases. Unhealthy habits can trickle down through generations, but it only takes one person to break the pattern. Fitness comes in all shapes and sizes...compare yourself only to your personal progress. The following page outlines some sample workouts for those new to exercise, especially suitable if you are 100 lb. or more overweight. Everyone has to start somewhere!

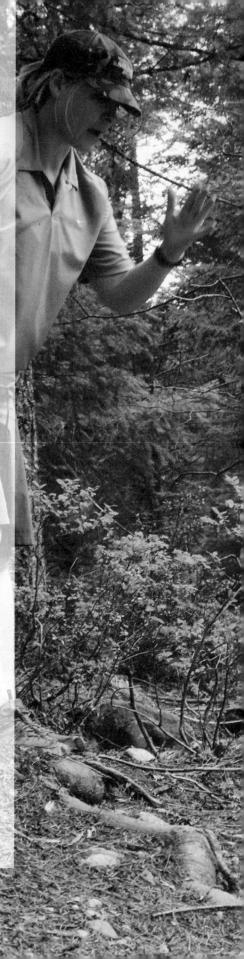

walking Intervals (pace should be based on heart rate) of 1-mile warm-up at a slow pace then stretch the lower body for 5 minutes, ¼ mile slow, ¼ mile medium, ¼ mile slow pace, 1 mile at fast pace.

If training on the treadmill, use a comfortable speed, adjusting the incline every few minutes. As you progress, start at a higher incline and go faster. Just be sure to keep your heart rate below 130 beats per minute, which is at a level that is still comfortable to talk. Knowing the shape of your feet is important and the gait of your running style.

Speak with a specialist who can analyze both your feet and gait, as they'll be able to recommend a good brand of shoe for you. Change your shoes every hundred miles run or walked to make sure they are still working for you.

step-ups Use a step (bench or box) that is approximately mid-shin height. Stand with both feet together and step up onto the box, finishing with both feet on top of the box; ensure the whole foot is on the box. Step back off the box and repeat using the other leg as the lead leg and alternate legs.

elliptical Mix up fat burning and cross-training mode to a maximum of 60 minutes, slow pace. Get your favorite music pumping and enjoy moving to the beats!

stationary bike Mix up random and hill mode to a maximum of 60 minutes, slow pace. Keep your heart rate monitored at all times and stay below 120 beats per minute. Start at comfortable RPM; aim to keep the same pace for the entire session. Every 4 weeks increase your RPM.

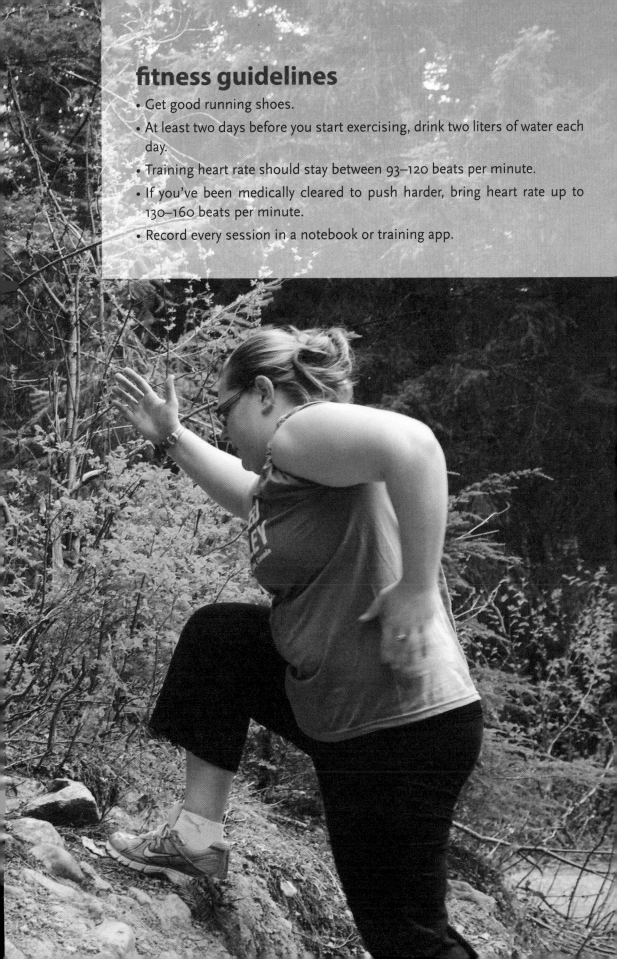

fitness guidelines

- Get good running shoes.
- At least two days before you start exercising, drink two liters of water each day.
- Training heart rate should stay between 93–120 beats per minute.
- If you've been medically cleared to push harder, bring heart rate up to 130–160 beats per minute.
- Record every session in a notebook or training app.

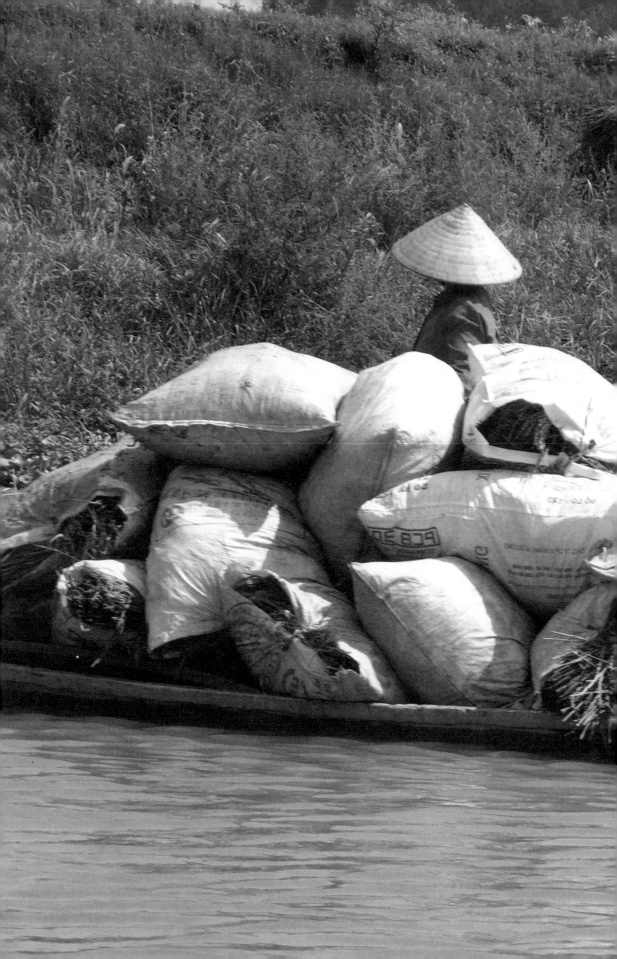

the planet friendly diet

how it works

The Planet Friendly Diet is about 1,200 calories per day — it's not advised to go lower than this. Plan snacks around personal preferences based on how many total calories you had that day. For example, Super Smoothies for breakfast (336 calories) and lunch (336 calories) then baked tilapia with lemon and coconut for dinner (330 calories) totals 1,002 calories, which means you can eat about 200 more calories on this day in snacks, like these below:

- Carrot sticks with salsa; you should end up with extra portions of homemade salsa now and then, so use this as an energizing low-calorie snack. This combination is high in vitamins A and C.

- Piece of fresh fruit: choose in-season varieties, like apples, pears and mandarins in winter; stone fruit, berries and melons in summer. If you have a juicer, you can refresh yourself with lots of delicious drinks. My best recipes are posted on catsmiley.com :)

- ½ cup of gluten-free cereal with low-fat non-dairy milk adds up to about 100 calories and will fill you up.

- Handful of unsalted pumpkin seeds — which is about 30 grams — equals about 120 calories. You'll find pumpkin seeds in the bulk bins at the grocery store.

- Tall non-dairy latte — my favorite — at about 120 calories, this milky coffee will fill you up when you're out and about with friends.

- 2 gluten-free rice cakes with hummus, alfalfa and thinly sliced red pepper. Mix it up with different homemade spreads, like tahini, yogurt-based dips and low-fat pesto. Try out new recipes; get creative.

how to make salsa

Salsa is the Spanish term for "sauce." To make 3 generous portions of 2–3 tablespoons per serving: chop up 2 large tomatoes, ½ jalapeño pepper, ½ bunch of cilantro, ¼ red onion and mix together in a bowl. Squeeze lemon juice over ingredients then refrigerate in storage container. If you're not a fan of cilantro, use parsley instead.

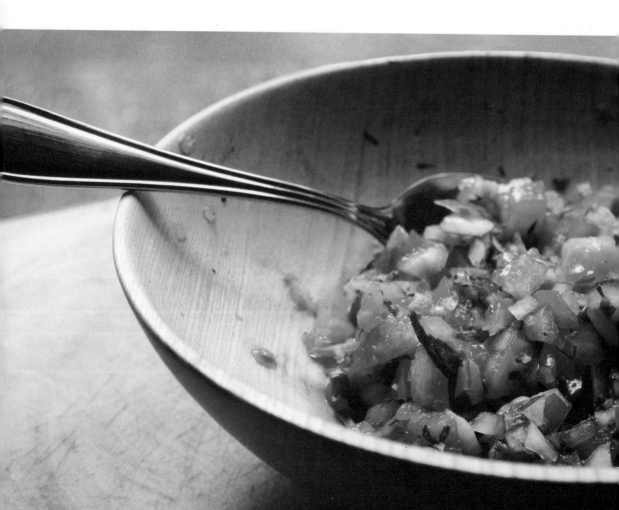

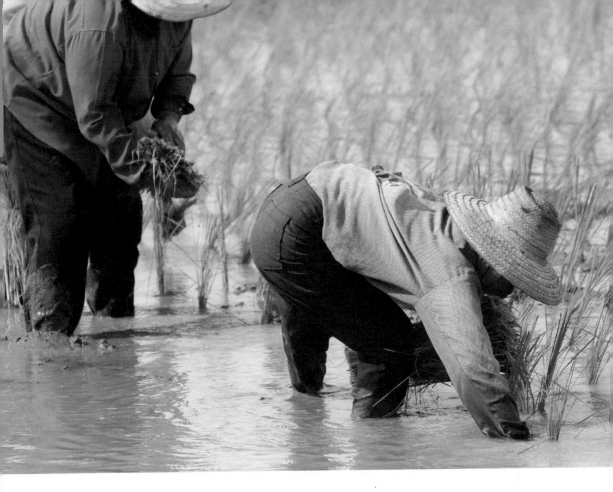

how to make rice

For light, fluffy grains, rinse rice in a large bowl of cold water first. Move rice around and pour out cloudy water. Repeat this step about 5 times, soak for 30 minutes, drain before starting the cooking process.

To make 2 cups of cooked rice: boil 2 cups of water in a pot, add ½ cup of uncooked rice and cook on low heat (with the lid on) for 30–40 minutes, stirring occasionally. Remove from heat, strain in sieve, rinse with warm water. Once cooled, transfer to storage container and refrigerate. This will make 4 regular portions. Some recipes call for 2 portions of rice, which is 1 cup cooked.

how to make vegetable broth

To make enough for 21 days, you will need: 6 large mushrooms, 3 stalks of celery, 2 medium carrots, 2 large leeks (white part only), 2 large tomatoes, 7 garlic cloves. Place vegetables on baking tray, roast in a 375°F/180°C oven until lightly brown. Boil 5 cups of water in a large pot.

Add roasted vegetables, cook at a low heat, covered, for 1 hour. Pour though a strainer into a storage container, refrigerate liquid once cooled. Make soup with the unused vegetables as a lunch alternative to the Super Smoothies.

At *Whistler Fitness Vacations*, we often use store-bought organic vegetable stock instead of making it from scratch. This is totally okay, as long as it's the low-sodium kind. The recipe is here for those of you who want to make everything yourself, or who don't have access to high-quality stock at your local grocery store.

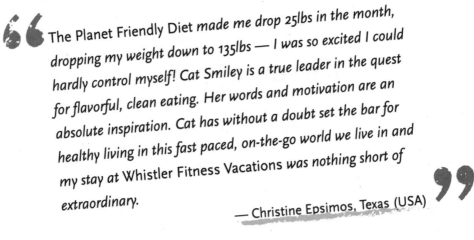

The Planet Friendly Diet *made me drop 25lbs in the month, dropping my weight down to 135lbs — I was so excited I could hardly control myself! Cat Smiley is a true leader in the quest for flavorful, clean eating. Her words and motivation are an absolute inspiration. Cat has without a doubt set the bar for healthy living in this fast paced, on-the-go world we live in and my stay at* Whistler Fitness Vacations *was nothing short of extraordinary.*

— Christine Epsimos, Texas (USA)

how to make super smoothies

Juicing is highly recommended if you can drink it within 15 minutes of making it, to ensure full antioxidant benefits. As we're away from the house all day at *Whistler Fitness Vacations*, we use this recipe.

Pour 1 cup almond milk and 2 cups water into a blender. Add 1 small frozen banana, 4 strawberries, handful of blueberries, 1 tablespoon non-dairy yogurt, handful of spinach and 1.5 scoops *Arbonne* protein powder (available at catsmiley.com). Mix on high for 10 seconds.

Your smoothie will be about 330 calories, based on the ingredient brands and quantity preferences that you're using. If you like it creamier, for example, add more non-dairy yogurt and reduce the milk alternative. Want it sweeter? Add more berries.

Adjust liquid measurements to suit personal preference. I blog my favorite smoothie and juicing recipes regularly at catsmiley. com

calories 336 | carbohydrates 52 g | protein 25 g | fat 4 g | estimated cost $2.25

beverages

Drink 4 liters of water a day — 2 liters before noon and 2 more liters before 5 pm. It seems like lots of water at first, but once you get used to it, you'll quickly see a boost in your energy levels and muscle recovery. Although water is not the only way to hydrate, it's the best. You'll boost your health and look much better too: clearer skin, shinier hair, fewer wrinkles!

the smoothie concept

The Planet Friendly Diet is a cleansing program designed to reset and replenish without fasting, hunger or deprivation. Due to the high level of physical activity at *Whistler Fitness Vacations*, traditional detoxification methods are not practical or safe. Toxins are materials that your body can't eliminate naturally through your digestive system — junk food, pollution, alcohol, drugs and so forth.

Antioxidants are substances that protect cells from the damage caused by unstable molecules known as free radicals. Examples of antioxidants include beta-carotene, lycopene and vitamins C and E. Many of these come from fruits and vegetables. Over the next 21 days, you'll eat between 7–13 servings of fruits and veggies per day, which is the recommended amount to protect against heart disease, certain types of cancers, obesity and type 2 diabetes.

For some people, this many servings seem like way too much sugar; however, keep in mind that sugars found in fruit (fructose) don't raise the blood sugar levels in the same way as refined or processed sugars. However, fruit contains over twice as much sugar content as vegetables, so if you're watching your insulin levels, lean more towards vegetables to hit the 7–13 quota. Ingredients for the Super Smoothies were selected based on berries being lower in natural sugars.

The shopping lists in this book are based on *Whistler Fitness Vacations* program of Super Smoothies for both breakfast and lunch. Ingredients are carefully designed to keep you energized and actually increase cravings for healthy foods. The low-fat blend of protein and carbohydrates helps to stabilize blood sugar levels and reduce appetite.

Super Smoothies are bursting with juicy berries, an endless array of other fresh ingredients, and a protein powder that blends smoothly without a strong taste. This powder provides enough high-quality protein to complement the carbohydrates and "good" fat, making smoothies the meal — not the meal replacement.

One of the benefits of smoothies is the shift in mindset; food becomes a non-event throughout the day, moving more towards being a function, or a necessity. Many guests find that this dramatically increases their excitement of the evening meal, as it's the one time that they get to savor the taste, relax, chew and enjoy!

Recent fructose research on the sugar content in fruit confirms that, despite its slower absorption rate than table sugars, the more sugar you eat, the more you will want — refined or natural. As many of my weight-loss clients come into my care with over 100 lb. to lose, loading them up with fruit often means severe side effects to follow when denied their cravings for chocolate and sweets.

We find that the breakfasts below provide a more gradual rise in blood glucose levels for those needing an alternative to doubling up the smoothies. If you're not a coffee drinker, enjoy with a cup of green tea! One study found that it not only boosts your metabolism, it also increases the speed at which your body burns fat.

alternative breakfast ideas

- ¼ cup (measured dry) cooked quinoa oatmeal with blueberries and almond or coconut milk
- 4 whipped egg whites made into an omelette with spinach, mushrooms, fresh salsa and 3 thinly sliced baby potatoes
- 1 cup gluten-free cereal (choose one with high protein) with baked apple, cinnamon and almond or coconut milk
- ½ cup (measured dry) oatmeal cooked with non-dairy milk and mango topped with cinnamon and a sprinkle of chopped almonds

alternative smoothie recipes

- 1 tablespoon peanut butter, 1 cup of coffee, 4 non-dairy chocolate milk cubes, 4 ice cubes, 1 small banana, ½ scoop protein powder, ½ cup non-dairy milk
- 1 small banana, 4 mango juice cubes, 4 strawberries, 2 coconut milk cubes, 1 tablespoon yogurt, water to taste, protein powder
- 1 small banana, handful of chopped pineapple, 4 orange juice cubes, 1 tablespoon yogurt, water to taste, ½ scoop protein powder
- ½ cup cranberries, 1 kiwi, 1 banana, water to taste, protein powder
- Juice of 1 orange, ½ mango, 4 slices pineapple, 1 cup coconut water, protein powder, 1 small banana, water to taste
- ½ bunch chopped spinach, juice of 2 limes, 4 slices pineapple, water to taste, ½ cup oatmeal, protein powder
- Juice of 3 oranges and 2 lemons, ½ cup fresh carrot juice, water to taste, 1 scoop protein powder

The measurement of protein powder depends on the brand that you are using. Figure it out to be at least 18g of protein. Find your favorite recipes by plugging them into an app on your smart phone, such as mynetdiary. com or similar. Be sure to get off to a good start with your daily fiber intake by including at least 5 grams with breakfast.

Going without solid food throughout the day is easier than you think, and is a powerful way to reset your metabolism. Numerous studies suggest that the human body evolved to perform at its best with short-term feeding gaps. Not only do insulin levels improve, it's also a fast and effective way to drop serious weight and change your behavior about food. From a religious sense, getting away from solid foods for a while can make you feel closer to your faith, as most people increase their prayer frequency in an effort to find strength, guidance and possibly forgiveness if they slip up by eating something they shouldn't have. If you are deciding to do intermittent fasting for spiritual or religious reasons, it's important that you arm yourself with minimal distractions — television, computer, smart phones — so that you can fully focus on increased prayer schedules and purifying your thoughts while you detoxify your body.

sunday shop, week 1

produce

14 small bananas,
1 large box strawberries and
1 large box blueberries, 7 lemons,
1 red onion, 1 garlic bulb,
1 small ginger root,
1–2 bunches spinach, 3 mushrooms,
2 portions broccoli, 3 portions green
beans, 2 large tomatoes, 1 jalapeño,
1 bunch cilantro (exchange with parsley if
you don't like cilantro),
1 yellow bell pepper,
2 red bell peppers, 1 cob corn,
1 zucchini, 1 small lettuce,
1 bag snow or snap peas, 1 carrot

deli

4 oz coconut crusted tilapia fillet,
3 oz white fish fillet, 4 oz sushi-grade ahi
tuna, 3 oz wild salmon,
1 package firm tofu,
250 g plain non-dairy yogurt,
2 liters non-dairy milk,
small block non-dairy cheese

frozen

1 bag lima beans
*frozen berries/corn if unavailable fresh

grocery

1 scoop dried black beans or organic can
1 kg brown rice
unsweetened coconut flakes
900 g vegan protein powder
1 packet paprika, coriander seed, cumin,
turmeric and chili spices,
sesame or chia seeds, 7 low-sugar snacks
of 100 cals (e.g., apples, pears,
gluten-free rice cakes,
hummus,
coconut water)

**budget
$110***
*Based on Whistler prices,
Nov 2015

some weeks

Check if you need plastic wrap, aluminum foil, paper towels, fresh spices, psyllium husk, fresh coffee and not forgetting delicious loose leaf tea for those late-night sweet treats after a day of planet friendly living. **Coconut crusted tilapia is a favorite at *Whistler Fitness Vacations,* but if it's not available, buy gluten-free bran flakes, rice flour and shredded unsweetened coconut flakes.

Every 21 days, buy 6 mushrooms, bunch of celery, garlic, 2 carrots, 2 large leeks and 2 large tomatoes extra to make broth.

when you get home

Make vegetable broth (page 24) if needed. Keep half in fridge, freeze remaining half. Peel bananas, wrap in plastic and store in the freezer. Wash berries, cut stalks off and freeze on a baking tray for a few hours, then move to storage container. Divide green beans into 3 servings and store in the fridge.

By the end of this week, you'll have left over: ½ yellow pepper, ½ jalapeño, some carrot and lettuce. Add these into recipes or have as snacks throughout the week.

Wrap fish fillets and freeze, place in fridge on the morning when needed. Cut tofu in half, freeze half and refridgerate half with the liquid in container. Empty rice into an airtight container.

Do you have your fabric bags?

day 1

baked tilapia with lemon and coconut (mexico)

There's so much flavor in this delicious dish, with its quick and easy crumb coating giving it just the right amount of carbs for day one on your kick-start. Remember, no salt allowed — it's delicious without!

1 clove garlic
3 oz tilapia fillet
3 mushrooms
4–5 broccoli florets
handful of green beans
1 teaspoon of paprika
2 tablespoons fresh salsa
½ lemon

For vegetarian option:
Cheese quesadilla, with whole grain tortilla. Place mushrooms inside with lightly cooked spinach and ¼ cup of black beans. Bake lightly, with 30 g of non-dairy cheese.

Preheat oven to 375°F/180°C.

If you have pre-seasoned fish, you're good to go. If you need to make the seasoning, mix ½ finely chopped red jalapeño, ½ cup non-dairy milk, 2 tablespoons crushed gluten-free cereal flakes, 1 tablespoon coconut flakes and 1 tablespoon rice flour in a bowl, then coat fish.

Place fish on aluminum foil, then bake for 15–20 minutes until fish is white when you put a knife through the centre.

While fish is cooking, make 3 portions of salsa (page 22) and put remainder in the fridge.

Slice mushrooms, chop broccoli, trim ends off beans. Peel, smash and chop garlic into fine pieces. Pour a few tablespoons of broth into a pan, simmer on medium heat until it bubbles.

Cook garlic and paprika until soft. Add mushrooms, broccoli and beans, cook until crisp. Serve with salsa and freshly squeezed lemon juice.

after dinner task:

- make 4 portions of rice (page 23)

calories 330 | carbohydrates 48 g | protein 27 g | fat 7 g
estimated cost $4.60

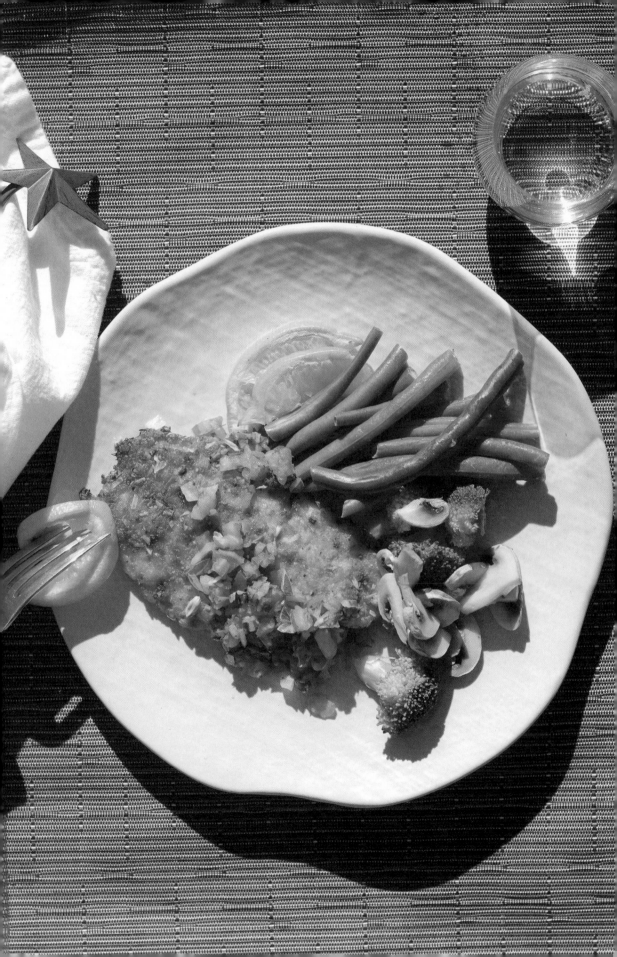

monday (sample)

weight: 178 lb.

goals:

- get through the day eating half as much as I normally do! OMG what have I got myself into!
- no chocolate after dinner
- no cookie with my chai latte when I meet Sarah at Starbucks
- complete day one of Cat's boot camp
- an hour of cardio
- figure out my heart rate monitor and calorie-tracking app
- no snack after dinner! herbal tea only!
- go to bed hungry

Below is an example of a perfect day on *The Planet Friendly Diet*. The "cost" is the amount of calories. Download an app like mynetdiary.com to keep within the guidelines.

Food	Cost	Time
breakfast super smoothie	336	8 am
snack rice cracker (gluten-free) with tablespoon of hummus, slice of red pepper and alfalfa	75	9:25 am
lunch super smoothie	336	11:30 am
snack double-shot soy latte, 12 oz	120	4 pm
dinner baked tilapia with lemon and coconut	330	6 pm

estimated calories eaten: 1,197   water: 4 liters

Reflection time! When you review your day, did you have any off-track moments, over-indulgences, emotional meltdowns or random acts of boredom eating that you regret? Use this space to write it down.

monday

weight:

goals:

notes:

Food	Cost	Time
breakfast		
snack		
lunch		
snack		
dinner		

estimated calories eaten: water:

day 2

colorful curry (india)

Tonight's meal will be love at first bite! India has inspired countries around the world to adapt a spice combination into their own cuisine. This bright summer dish is rich and creamy, perfect for beginners to put together.

1 clove garlic
1 teaspoon of turmeric, cumin and coriander seeds
1 tablespoon coconut flakes
3 oz white fish
handful of green beans
½ yellow bell pepper
½ cob of corn
½ cup cooked rice
½ cup non-dairy milk
1 tablespoon non-dairy yogurt

For vegetarian option: Sautéed cauliflower and high-protein non-dairy yogurt or cottage cheese, mixed with a tablespoon of seeds.

Preheat oven to 375°F/180°C and boil a pot of water. Place fish on aluminum foil, and cook in preheated oven, for 15–20 minutes. When water is boiled, add corn to pot and cook until bright yellow. This will take about 6 minutes, so while you wait, peel, smash and chop garlic, cut the ends off beans and slice pepper.

Remove corn from pot and rinse in cold water. Break in half and remove kernels in downwards slicing motion on a chopping board.

Pour generous amount of broth into a pan and cook over medium heat, until it bubbles. Add garlic, coconut flakes and spices; sauté for a few minutes then add beans, corn, yellow pepper. After a few minutes, add rice to the pan.

Check fish — if it is white when you put a knife through the centre, it is ready. Add to the pan. Pour non-dairy milk over ingredients and simmer gently for 3 minutes on medium heat. Add more spices to taste, serve with dollop of yogurt and your favorite Bollywood movie!

calories 388 | carbohydrates 53 g | protein 27 g | fat 4 g
estimated cost $2.95

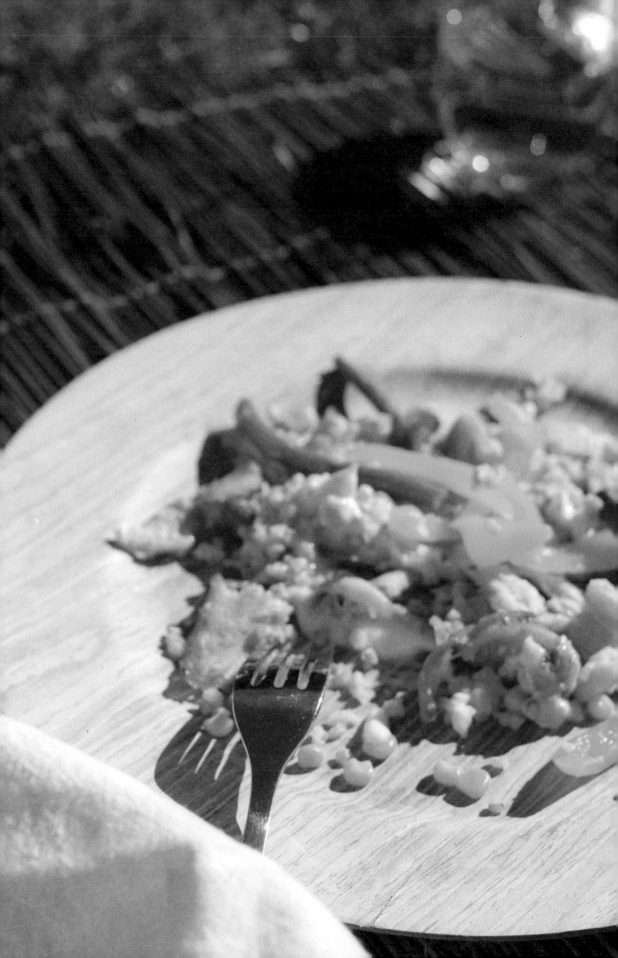

tuesday

weight:

goals:

notes:

Food	Cost	Time
breakfast		
snack		
lunch		
snack		
dinner		

estimated calories eaten: water:

day 3

ahi steak with spicy rice (costa rica)

The secret of seared steak is to let it marinate for just the right amount of time — for fish, 20 minutes is tops. This dish is meaty and flavorful, popular for people missing their land animals.

¼ small onion
1 clove garlic
1 teaspoon of sesame seeds
sprinkle of chili powder
1 teaspoon of paprika
1 lemon
4–5 broccoli florets
1 handful of spinach
¼ red bell pepper
4 oz ahi tuna
½ cup cooked brown rice
2 tablespoons salsa

For vegetarian option: Whole grain quinoa, ½ cob of corn and scrambled tofu. Make it Gallo Pinto by adding cilantro, garlic and onion — skip the broccoli.

Fill bowl with juice from squeezed lemon and soak tuna in it for 15 minutes. Get the most out of the lemon by sticking a fork in it and twisting until fully juiced.

Cut stems off spinach. Chop broccoli, garlic and onion. Slice red pepper.

Pour a few tablespoons of broth into a pan and cook over medium heat until it bubbles. Add onion, garlic, paprika and chili spices to pan, cook until tender. Add broccoli and red pepper, cook until crispy, remove from heat and mix with raw spinach.

Place rice in pan, stirring with wooden spoon until very hot. Preheat new pan, pour in broth to taste and cook tuna in bubbling liquid for 2 minutes on each side, until lightly crusted. The inside will stay pink, but if it is too undercooked for you, bake at 375°F/180°C for 10 minutes before searing.

Top with sesame seeds and serve with the salsa made on day 1.

calories 373 | carbohydrates 61 g | protein 30 g | fat 2.5 g
estimated cost $4.95

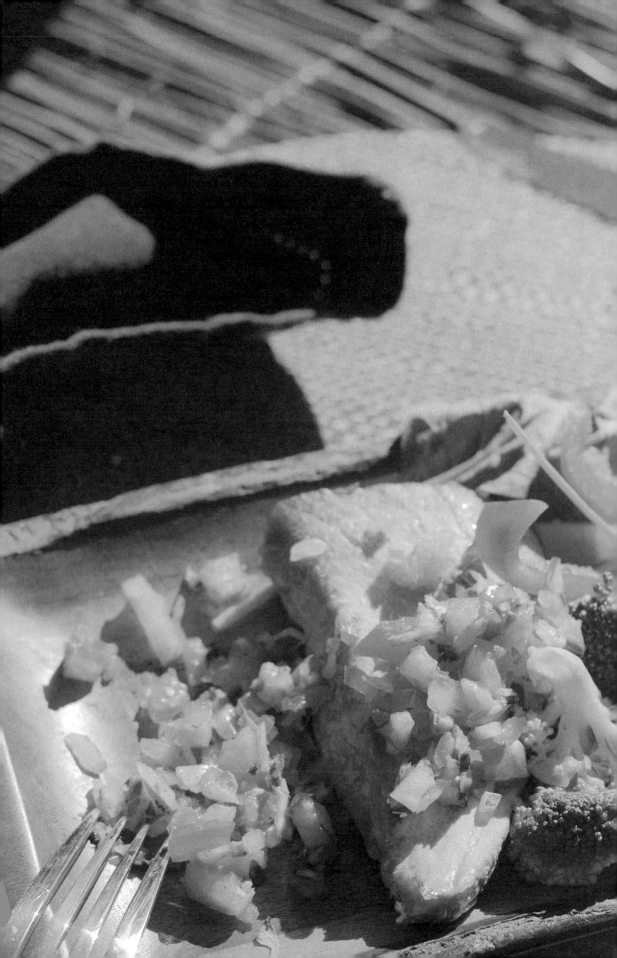

wednesday

weight:

goals:

notes:

Food	Cost	Time
breakfast		
snack		
lunch		
snack		
dinner		

estimated calories eaten: water:

day 4

festive tofu curry (indonesia)

High in protein, this vibrant meal will wake up your senses, leaving you energized with its big kick of flavor. Whether it's crazy-hot or mild and creamy, you'll get addicted to curry in a hurry with this kick-ass blend of spices.

1 teaspoon of turmeric, cumin and coriander
¼ package firm tofu
¼ red bell pepper
handful of green beans
handful of snap peas
½ cup non-dairy milk
½ cup cooked brown rice
1 tablespoon non-dairy yogurt

Chop tofu into small cubes, slice red pepper, cut ends off snap peas. Pour a few tablespoons of broth into a pan and cook over medium heat until it bubbles.

Add tofu and spices and fry at medium heat until all sides are crispy. Add bell pepper, green beans and snap peas. Pour non-dairy milk over vegetables and add rice to pan (cooked on Day 1).

Play with the spices — make it as hot as you can handle, then cool it down with a dollop of non-dairy yogurt while letting your mind travel to the warm waves of Bali....

after dinner task:

- wash 3.5 cups of black beans, soak overnight in 10 cups of water. Tomorrow cook beans for 2 hours before dinner.

calories 392 | carbohydrates 67 g | protein 23 g | fat 8 g
estimated cost $2.80

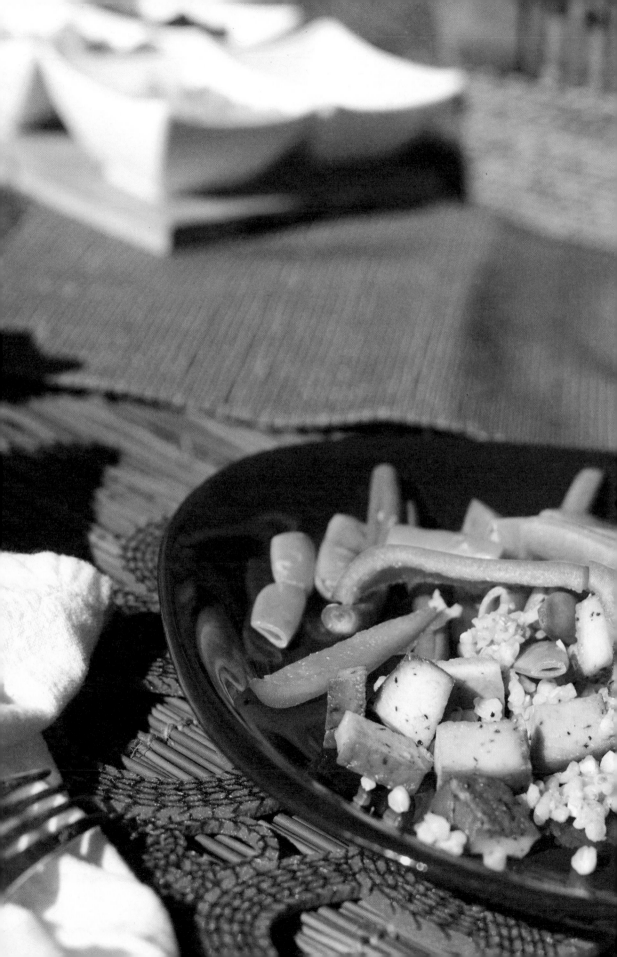

thursday

weight:

goals:

notes:

Food	Cost	Time
breakfast		
snack		
lunch		
snack		
dinner		

estimated calories eaten: water:

day 5

tex-mex stuffed pepper (mexico)

This is a favorite for hungry families around the world; not only tasty, but nutritionally well-balanced too.

¼ onion
1 clove garlic
1 teaspoon of paprika
sprinkle of chili powder
½ cob of corn
½ zucchini
1 red bell pepper
½ cup lima beans
¼ cup cooked black beans
¼ cup cooked brown rice
30 g non-dairy cheese
2 leaves iceberg lettuce
2 tablespoons salsa

You'll need to start prep for tonight's meal a few hours before dinner because the beans need to cook. Simmer the soaked beans for 2 hours on low heat, adding more water every 30 minutes or so if needed.

Preheat oven to 350°F. Cook lima beans and corn for 6 minutes in a pot of boiling water until bright and tender. Rinse under cold water, break corn in half and remove kernels in downwards slicing motion. Peel and chop garlic. Chop onion finely.

Pour a few tablespoons of broth into a pan and cook over medium heat until it bubbles. Add spices, onion, garlic and zucchini. Stir with wooden spoon, until tender. Add lima beans, black beans, cooked rice and corn to pan. Cook for 3 minutes. Cut top off pepper, remove seeds and stuff with mixture. Grate cheese (about 2 tablespoons) on top, bake until melted.

Serve with lettuce and salsa. You will have salsa in the fridge from day 1.

after dinner tasks:

- transfer remaining black beans to tray and freeze. Move to storage container when frozen.

- make 2 portions of rice (page 23)

calories 418 | carbohydrates 42 g | protein 22 g | fat 9 g
estimated cost $2.50

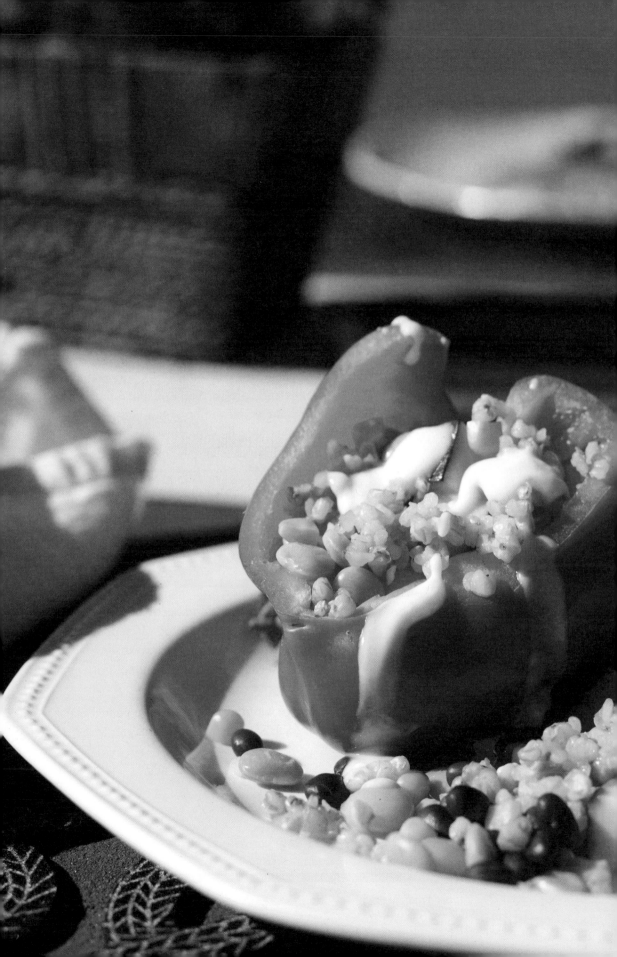

friday

weight:

goals:

notes:

Food	Cost	Time
breakfast		
snack		
lunch		
snack		
dinner		

estimated calories eaten: water:

day 6

baked salmon with spinach salad (canada)

Salmon is one of the most loved dishes of the Pacific Northwest, from Vancouver up to Alaska; the bright pink color stands out at the fish market like a fabulous friend. This recipe is made to impress!

1 inch ginger root
1 teaspoon of cumin
½ lemon
1–2 sprigs cilantro
3 oz wild salmon
½ zucchini
handful of snap peas
1 cup cooked brown rice
½ small carrot
handful of spinach

For vegetarian option: Substitute salmon with seitan (also known as wheat gluten), a specialty item with great texture and meat-like protein.

Preheat oven to 350°F/180°C. Prepare fish by squeezing lemon over the fillet and placing it on aluminum foil.

Cut ends off snap peas, slice zucchini, chop spinach. Chop cilantro finely. Peel ginger and chop into fine pieces. Pour a few tablespoons of broth into a pan and cook over medium heat until it bubbles. Add cilantro, ginger and spices, then zucchini and snap peas. Cook until tender. Add rice. Stir with a wooden spoon for a few minutes on high heat.

For the salad, peel and grate carrot, mix into raw spinach. Dress with freshly squeezed lemon juice. Check the salmon after 15–20 minutes. Put the tip of the knife into the center — it should be pale pink inside.

Serve with ground pepper to taste, but remember, no salt!

calories 393 | carbohydrates 57 g| protein 29 g | fat 6 g
estimated cost $4.85

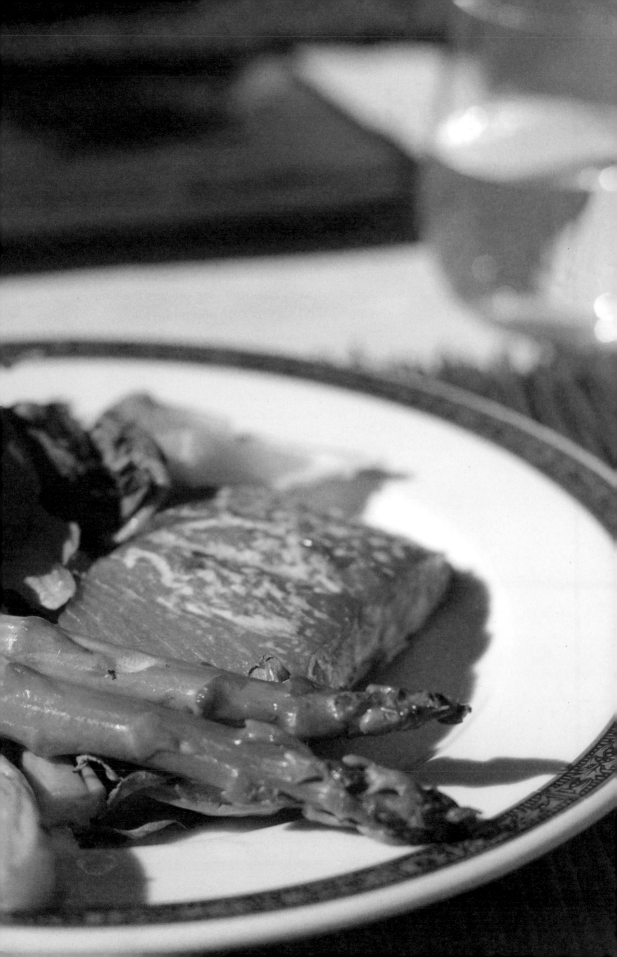

saturday

weight:

goals:

notes:

Food	Cost	Time
breakfast		
snack		
lunch		
snack		
dinner		

estimated calories eaten: water:

day 7

arroz con frijoles (argentina)

This Latin American favorite is famous for its simplicity and natural flavors; the sweet bell pepper and fresh lettuce blend beautifully with rich cheese, delicious with homemade salsa. This sauce, which can be traced to the Aztecs, Mayans and Incas, was officially named "salsa" in 1571.

1 clove garlic
1 teaspoon of paprika
1 teaspoon of chili powder
¼ bunch cilantro
½ red bell pepper
½ cup cooked black beans
2 leaves iceberg lettuce
½ cup cooked brown rice
30 g non-dairy cheese
2 tablespoons salsa
¼ lemon
pepper

Slice bell pepper and chop lettuce. Peel, smash and chop garlic. Make 3 portions of salsa (page 22) and put what you don't use tonight into the fridge.

Pour a few tablespoons of broth into a pan and cook over medium heat until it bubbles. Add spices, fry at medium heat.

Stir bell pepper into pan, add rice and beans, cook for a few minutes stirring occasionally with wooden spoon.

Arrange lettuce on a plate and top with cooked food. Grate cheese (about 2 tablespoons) onto meal. Serve with salsa. For extra zest, add lemon juice and sprinkle cracked pepper to taste.

after dinner tasks:

- grocery shop for next week
- Make 1½ cups cooked quinoa. Rinse and strain ¼ cup dry grain under cold running water, place in 2 cups boiling water. Cook 20 minutes on low heat. Refrigerate in container.

calories 421 | carbohydrates 75 g | protein 20 g | fat 6.5 g
estimated cost $1.80

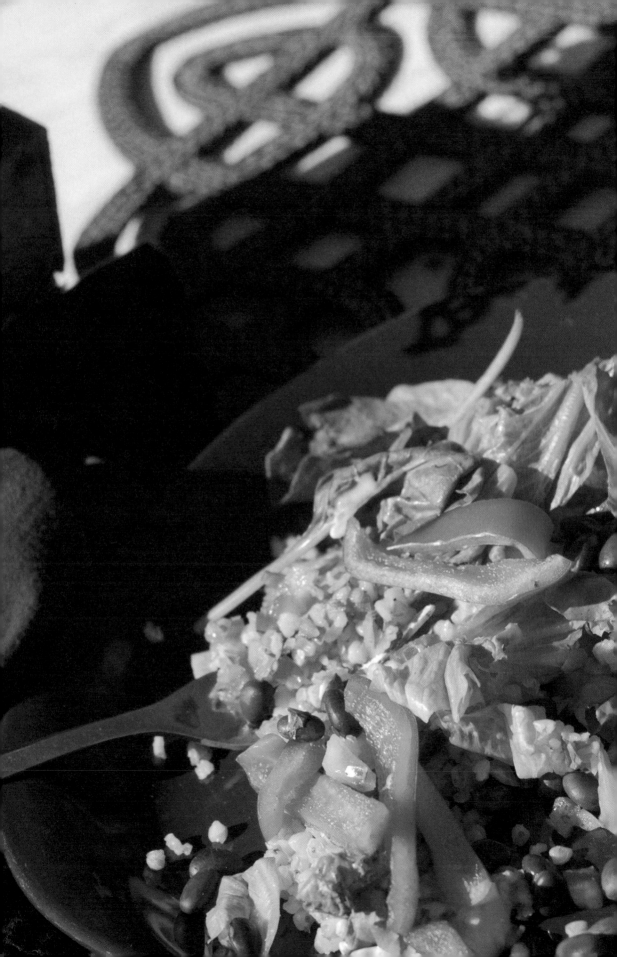

sunday

weight:

goals:

notes:

Food	Cost	Time
breakfast		
snack		
lunch		
snack		
dinner		

estimated calories eaten: water:

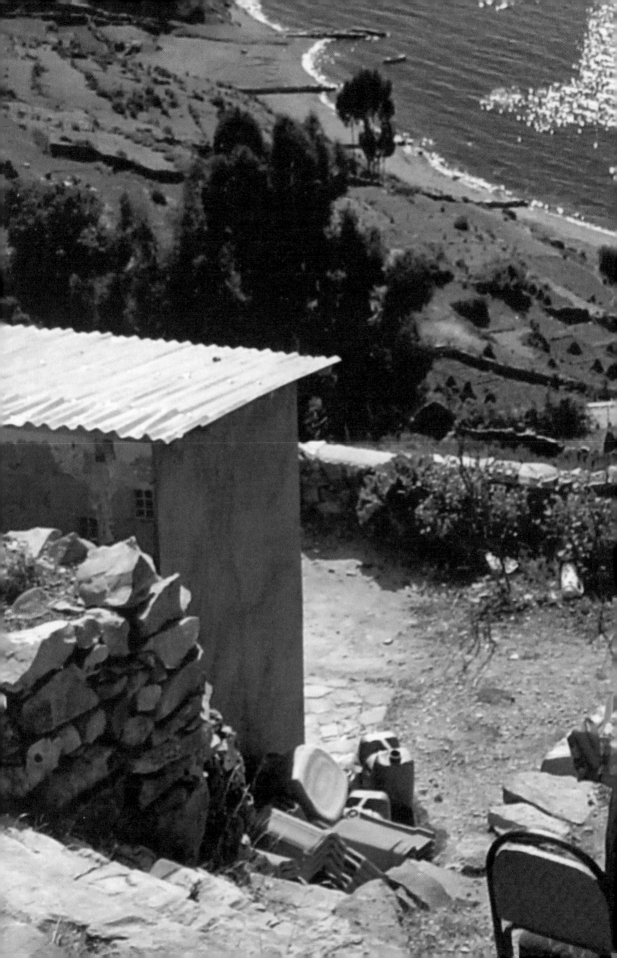

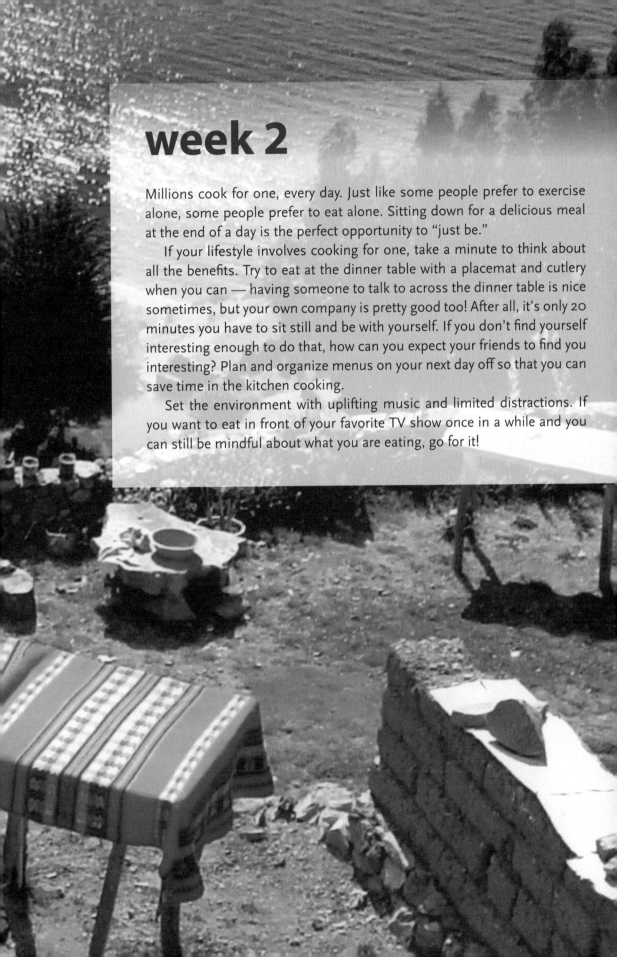

week 2

Millions cook for one, every day. Just like some people prefer to exercise alone, some people prefer to eat alone. Sitting down for a delicious meal at the end of a day is the perfect opportunity to "just be."

If your lifestyle involves cooking for one, take a minute to think about all the benefits. Try to eat at the dinner table with a placemat and cutlery when you can — having someone to talk to across the dinner table is nice sometimes, but your own company is pretty good too! After all, it's only 20 minutes you have to sit still and be with yourself. If you don't find yourself interesting enough to do that, how can you expect your friends to find you interesting? Plan and organize menus on your next day off so that you can save time in the kitchen cooking.

Set the environment with uplifting music and limited distractions. If you want to eat in front of your favorite TV show once in a while and you can still be mindful about what you are eating, go for it!

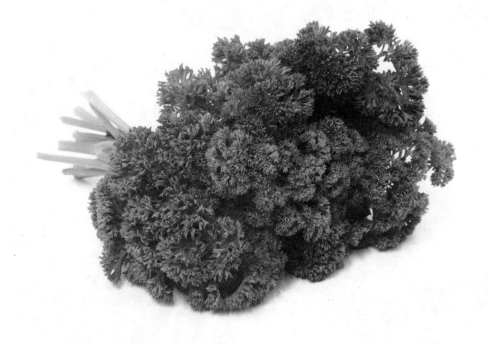

sunday shop, week 2

produce

14 small bananas
650 g strawberries
large box blueberries
2 + lemons
small bag green beans
small bag snap peas
½ cup edamame beans
1 green bell pepper
1 orange bell pepper
8 small potatoes
1 bunch asparagus
1 cob of corn
1 head of celery
1 portion broccoli
small iceberg lettuce
1 avocado
3 tomatoes
1 bunch of spinach
handful of bean sprouts
½ red cabbage
1 red jalapeño pepper

deli

4 oz wild salmon
1 tub non-dairy yogurt

grocery

185 g tin light tuna
tin of organic baby corn
20 unsalted almonds
12 unsalted blanched peanuts
1 packet of rosemary
1 scoop of quinoa grains
1 can organic black beans (if you
didn't cook them last week)

when you get home

Peel bananas, wrap, store in freezer.
Wash produce. Cut tops off strawberries
and freeze on a baking tray with the
blueberries. Keeping them separate on
a tray means they won't stick together,
transfer to a storage container once
frozen.

Divide green beans into 2 servings
and refrigerate. You only need 1 serving
of snap peas and ¾ of the green pepper;
they won't keep so add them to any
meal or enjoy as a snack. Do the same
with extra celery.

Cut tofu into quarters and freeze
¾ of package. You already have some
in the freezer but need more for the
upcoming week — use the oldest
first. After Day 8, use up the rest of the
baby corn in any meal. Save half the
almonds for next week. Make quinoa —
instructions on day 7.

Do you have your fabric bags?

budget
$60*
*Based on Whistler prices,
Nov 2015

day 8

edamame energizer (japan)

Japan has the lowest obesity rate in the developed world — their diet is clean and nutritionally balanced. In a land that accounts for just 2% of the world's population, its people eat 10% of the world's seafood — so when they take a night off from fish, they do it to perfection!

1 clove garlic
1 inch ginger root
1 tablespoon sesame seeds
½ lemon
½ tomato
½ cup red cabbage
* ½ cup edamame beans
handful of bean sprouts
handful of spinach
½ cup cooked quinoa

* Option: use lima beans.

Boil pot of water and cook ½ cup edamame in shells for 6 minutes. Rinse under cold water once cooked and remove from shells.

Chop cabbage and cut tomato into thin slices, cut stems off spinach. Peel, smash and chop both garlic and ginger finely. Pour a few tablespoons of broth into a pan and cook over medium heat until it bubbles. Fry garlic and ginger in pan. Squeeze lemon juice into mixture.

Add sesame seeds — jiggle pan so that they can spread out and lightly brown without burning. Stir with a wooden spoon.

Add cabbage, spinach and quinoa to the pan; cook for 2 minutes, then mix edamame, bean sprouts and tomato into the cooked ingredients. Squeeze fresh lemon juice, break out the chopsticks and enjoy! This dish is great hot or cold.

after dinner task:
- cook ½ cup dry rice with 1 cup water (page 23). Refrigerate in container.

calories 421 | carbohydrates 56 g | protein 26 g | fat 12 g
estimated cost $2.20

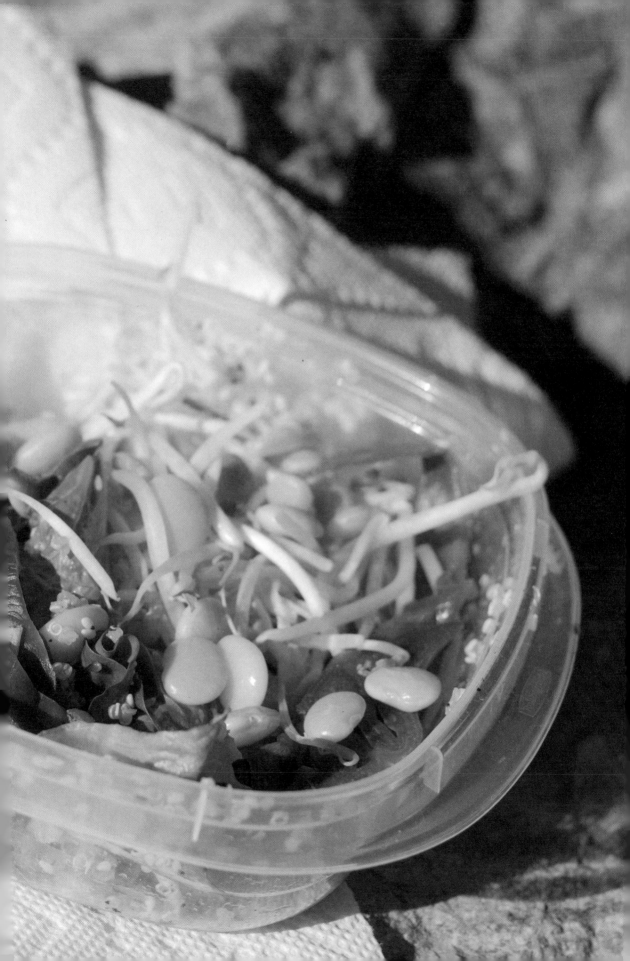

monday

weight:

goals:

notes:

Food	Cost	Time
breakfast		
snack		
lunch		
snack		
dinner		

estimated calories eaten: water:

day 9

gado-gado (indonesia)

You'll go nuts for this Southeast Asian classic, a popular choice for stir-fry cooking with its flavorful, mellow twist. This versatile sauce can also be used in the curry dishes.

1 clove garlic
1 ginger root
handful of green beans
4–5 pieces broccoli
¼ orange bell pepper
½ can baby corn
½ package of firm tofu
1 cup cooked brown rice
½ cup non-dairy milk
12 blanched peanuts
1 teaspoon of turmeric
sprinkle of chili powder
lemon slices

Peel, smash and chop both garlic and ginger into fine pieces.

To make the peanut sauce: pour a few tablespoons of broth into a pan and cook over medium heat until it bubbles. Add garlic, ginger and spices, fry at medium heat. Place peanuts in plastic wrap and crush with end of cutting knife. Add crushed peanuts, toast until tender, jiggling pan to avoid burning. Remove from heat and put mixture into blender with non-dairy milk. You might need to add some water. Blend on high until grainy and smooth. If you have some coconut left over from last week, add a tablespoon or so.

Wash corn extra well to remove any additional salt. Add vegetables and tofu to the pan, cook with peanut sauce for a few minutes, stirring occasionally. Serve with non-dairy yogurt and lemon.

calories 435 | carbohydrates 75 g | protein 20 g | fat 6 g
estimated cost $2.90

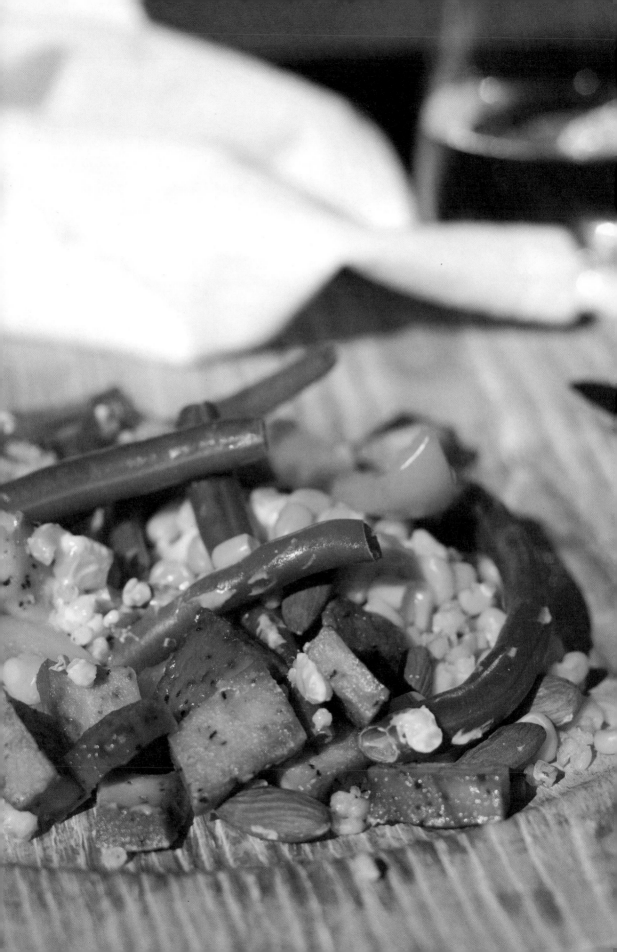

tuesday

weight:

goals:

notes:

Food	Cost	Time
breakfast		
snack		
lunch		
snack		
dinner		

estimated calories eaten: water:

day 10

simple salmon (canada)

Salmon is the star of this recipe, but wait till you meet its sidekicks! Oven-roasted asparagus has intense, delicate flavors that blend beautifully with the bite-size potatoes.

1 teaspoon of rosemary
4 oz wild salmon
6 spears asparagus
5 potatoes
1 lemon

For vegetarian option: Substitute salmon with chickpea burger, with spicy Greek yogurt and fresh tomato. Reduce potato serving, as the chickpeas are enough carb.

Preheat oven to 375°F/180°C.

Bring a pot of water to the boil, add potatoes, cook for 8 to 10 minutes until soft. Chop into bite-size pieces.

Trim ends of asparagus.

Place salmon, asparagus and potatoes on baking tray lined with aluminum foil. Sprinkle rosemary over potatoes, drizzle lemon juice over salmon and roast in oven for 20 minutes. If you have some red onion in the fridge, chop up a few slices and cook with the salmon.

The fish is cooked when the center is pale pink — check with a fork — the asparagus and potatoes only need about 10 minutes tops in the oven.

calories 377 | carbohydrates 46 g | protein 33 g | fat 8 g
estimated cost $4.75

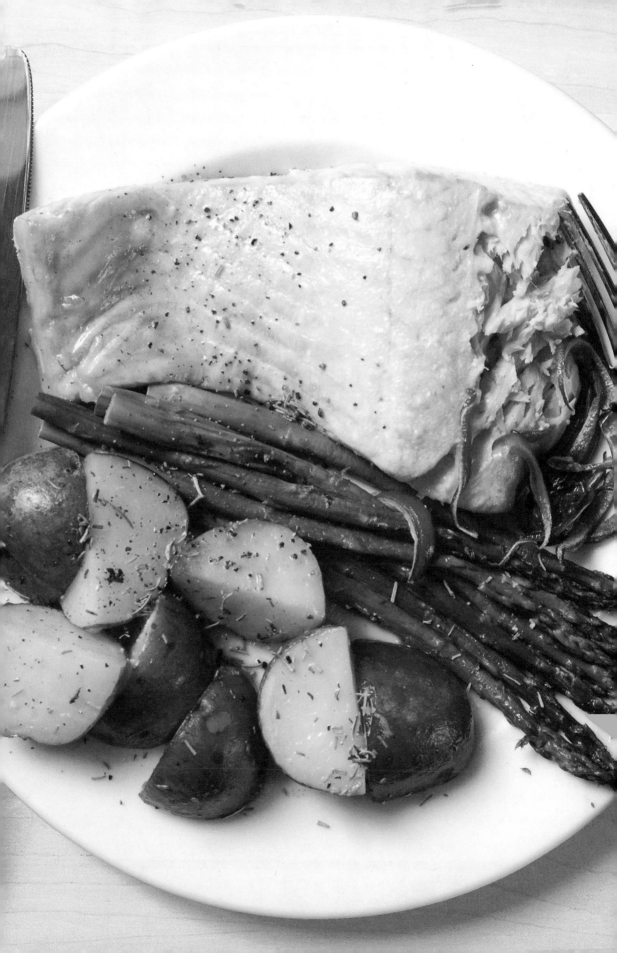

wednesday

weight:

goals:

notes:

Food	Cost	Time
breakfast		
snack		
lunch		
snack		
dinner		

estimated calories eaten: water:

day 11

wonder bean quinoa (peru)

Quinoa (keen-wa) has been an important food in South America for over 6,000 years — the Incas called it "the Mother of all Grains." Full of vitality and vitamins, this sunny dish is awesome for days you need an extra boost.

1 teaspoon of paprika
pinch of chili powder
¼ jalapeño pepper
½ cup lima beans
1 cob of corn
1 sprig of cilantro
10 unsalted almonds
1 lemon
1 cup cooked quinoa
¼ tomato

Boil a pot of water, cook lima beans and corn for 6 minutes. Rinse under cold water, break corn in half and remove kernels with a downwards slicing motion.

Chop cilantro and jalapeño pepper finely. Pour a few tablespoons of broth into a pan and cook over medium heat, until it bubbles. Add cilantro, jalapeño pepper, chili powder and paprika; fry on medium heat.

Add almonds and cooked quinoa to pan, stir with wooden spoon once or twice and cook for a few minutes. Remove from heat, mix all ingredients together. Squeeze lemon, add juice and serve with finely chopped tomato or salsa.

Enjoy hot or cold.

calories 469 | carbohydrates 69 g | protein 22 g | fat 13 g
estimated cost $3.10

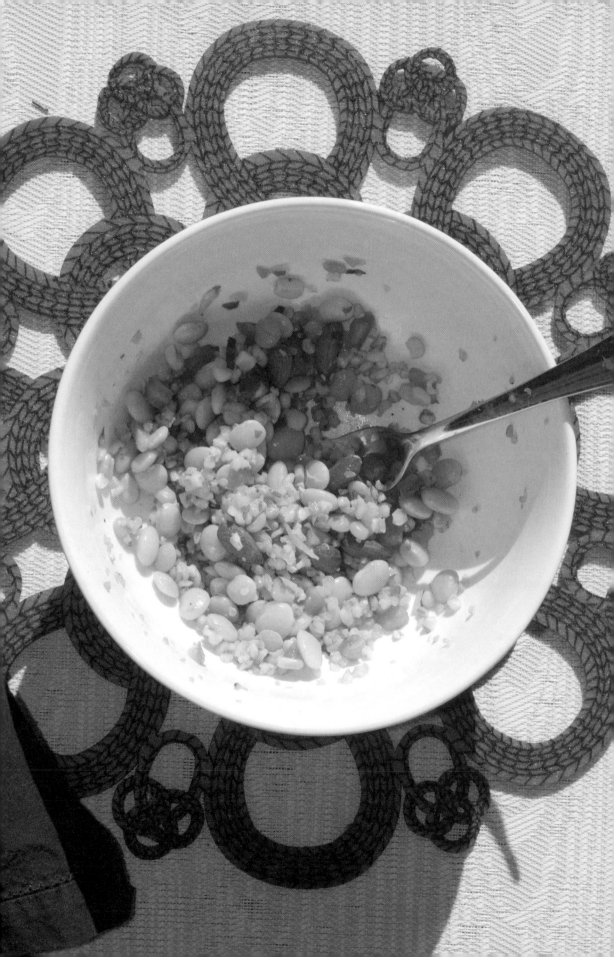

thursday

weight:

goals:

notes:

Food	Cost	Time
breakfast		
snack		
lunch		
snack		
dinner		

estimated calories eaten: water:

day 12

neesuaz tuna salad (france)

It's amazing how much a salad can fill you up. This dish is a spin on the Niçoise (pronounced nee-suaz) salad which originated from Nice in the Mediterranean. It's a lighter version of the American cobb salad with tuna, beans and potato, packed with muscle-building protein. Yum!

1 clove garlic
1 teaspoon of turmeric
1 teaspoon of paprika
pinch of chili powder
1 can light tuna
handful of green beans
¼ green bell pepper
3 small new potatoes
¼ avocado
½ tomato
1 stalk celery
1 sprig cilantro
2 tablespoons yogurt
¼ head iceberg lettuce
30 g soy cheese

Boil a pot of water, cook potatoes for 5–8 minutes. Slice green pepper, avocado, celery and tomato. Cut ends off beans. Peel, smash and chop garlic. Chop cilantro finely. Cut potatoes into bite-size pieces. Drain can of tuna.

Pour a few tablespoons of broth into a pan and cook over medium heat until it bubbles. Fry garlic and turmeric, add potatoes, cook until lightly crisp. With a fork, mix tuna in a large bowl with celery, cilantro and yogurt.

Grate cheese and mix it in a bowl with raw vegetables, tuna, potatoes and cooked spicy garlic.

Prepare lettuce bowl by hitting the cut end of the lettuce on the kitchen counter to remove core. Take off about 2 outer leaves.

Assemble salad into lettuce bowl, garnish with paprika or chili.

For vegetarian option:
Substitute tuna with scrambled tofu or egg whites.

after dinner tasks:

- make 2 portions of rice (page 23)
- move 1 portion black beans from freezer to fridge
- defrost vegetable broth

calories 455 | carbohydrates 51 g | protein 36 g | fat 15 g
estimated cost $3.90

80 | *The Planet Friendly Diet*

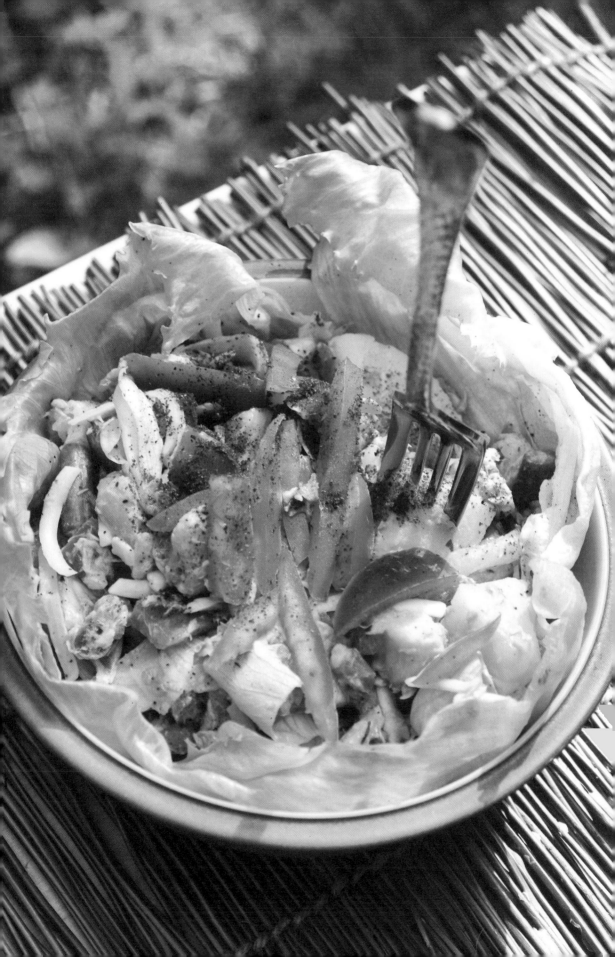

friday

weight:

goals:

notes:

Food	Cost	Time
breakfast		
snack		
lunch		
snack		
dinner		

estimated calories eaten: water:

day 13

el cheapo (jamaica)

Basic beans and rice bursting with flavor — a modern combo of raw and cooked foods, full of natural hot spices. Bob Marley said, "Love the life you live, live the life you love." Bringing plates of happiness to the dinner table will help you do just that!

1 clove garlic
1 teaspoon of paprika
pinch of chili powder
¼ avocado
¼ red jalapeño pepper
¼ cup cooked black beans
2 leaves iceberg lettuce
½ orange bell pepper
½ tablespoon lemon juice
¼ package tofu
½ cup cooked brown rice

Drain excess water from tofu, cut into small cubes. Chop garlic, jalapeño and lettuce leaves and slice orange pepper. Peel avocado.

Pour a few tablespoons of broth into a pan and cook over medium heat until it bubbles. Add paprika, garlic and jalapeño; fry at medium with chili powder. Add tofu. Cook until crispy. Mix in rice and beans, let simmer until hot. Stir gently with wooden spoon to avoid burning.

Pour lemon juice over raw ingredients and assemble on a plate with cooked ingredients.

calories 445 | carbohydrates 55 g | protein 23 g | fat 18 g
estimated cost $1.55

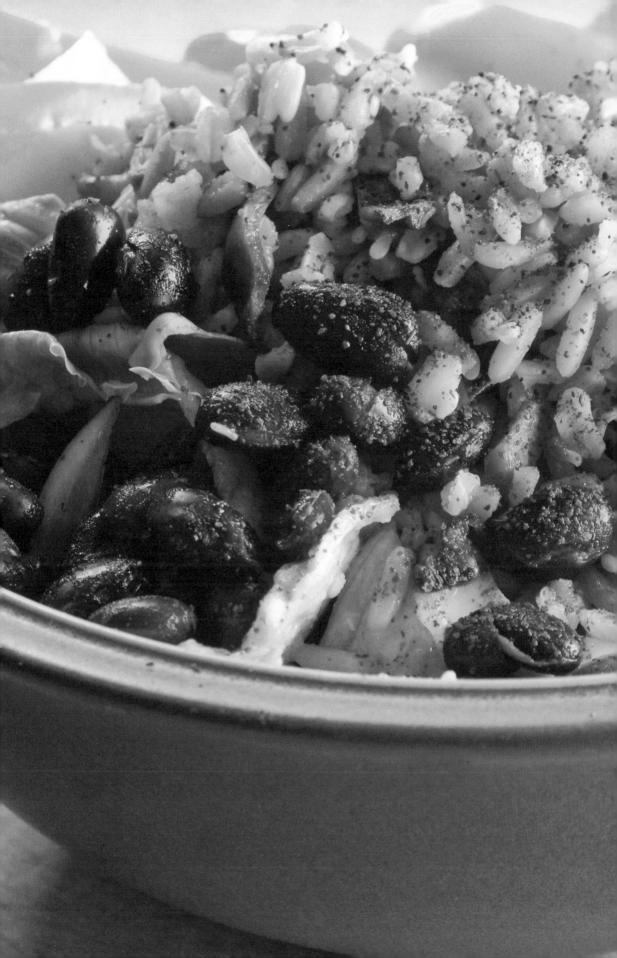

saturday

weight:

goals:

notes:

Food	Cost	Time
breakfast		
snack		
lunch		
snack		
dinner		

estimated calories eaten: water:

day 14

sesame stir-fry (hong kong)

Challenge yourself to embrace another vegan day! You'll love the sweet taste of ginger and crunchy sesame seeds as they ooze into the silky tofu and punch out this healthy stir-fry. Snap peas give that delicate green crunch, while the red cabbage is a vegetable lover's delight.

1 inch ginger root
1 teaspoon of coriander
1 teaspoon of cumin
1 tablespoon sesame seeds
¼ package tofu
½ cup red cabbage
¼ orange bell pepper
handful of snap peas
½ cup cooked brown rice

Trim ends off snap peas, slice bell pepper, chop cabbage. Cut tofu into cubes. Peel, smash and chop ginger finely.

Pour a few tablespoons of broth into a pan and cook over medium heat until it begins to bubble. Add ginger and spices and fry. Add sesame seeds — jiggle pan to spread out and lightly brown without burning. Add tofu, fry until crisp then add cabbage, orange pepper and snap peas. You might need to add more liquid. Cook until softened but still crispy. Add rice and let cook for 5 minutes.

after dinner task:

- grocery shopping

calories 403 | carbohydrates 58 g | protein 20 g | fat 10.5 g
estimated cost $2.00

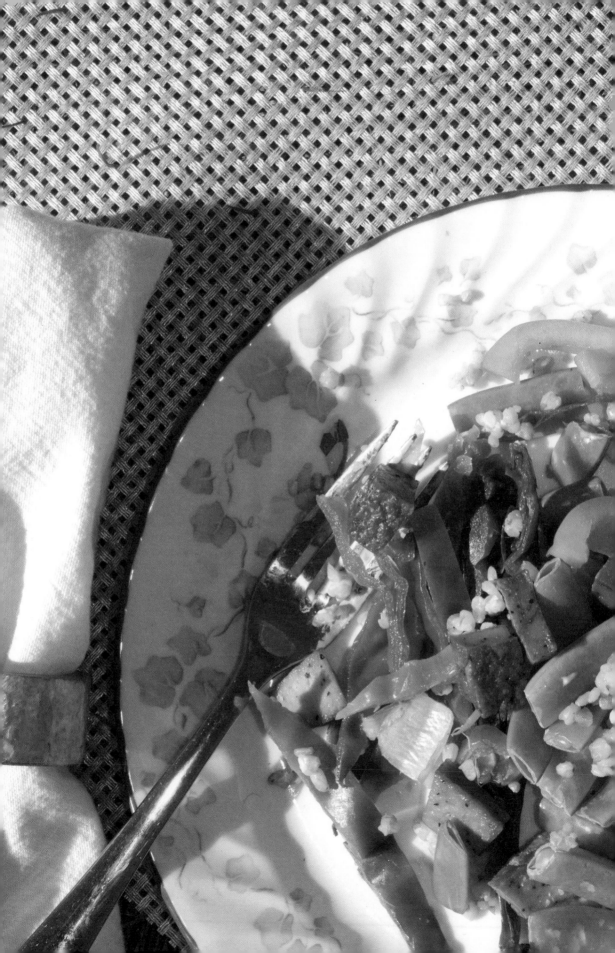

sunday

weight:

goals:

notes:

Food	Cost	Time
breakfast		
snack		
lunch		
snack		
dinner		

estimated calories eaten: water:

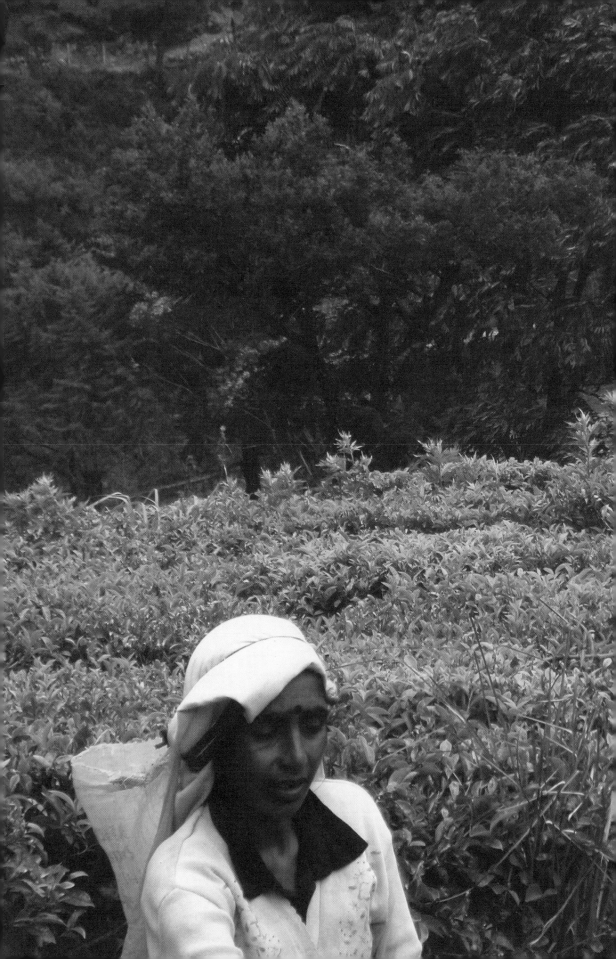

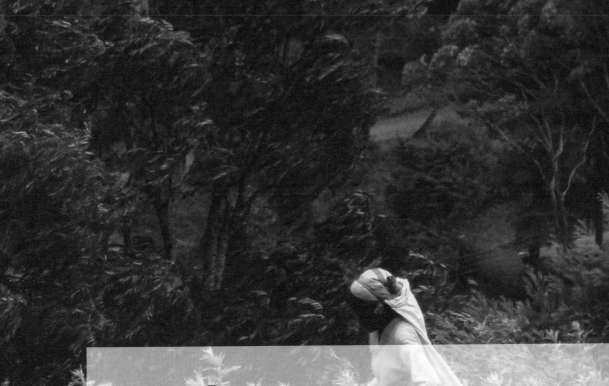

week 3

Breaking up is hard to do — even if it's with your food habits. But just as certain foods can cause headaches, so can certain changes in your diet. Before reaching for medication, try to sit for a few moments and relax, meditate... just be. You're doing great, don't stress or worry about things too much. Breathe through some positive affirmations to reclaim your awesome. If that doesn't work, take a hot shower (warm water can relax your muscles), sit down in a quiet place, put your feet up, put a bag of frozen peas on your head and drink water. You may be behind on your water quota today, which could be causing headaches. Have an espresso — caffeine is a key ingredient in painkillers. If you're not into coffee, opt for green tea. Power nap, rest your brain. You may be sleep deprived. Eat a green apple. Chew slowly... a natural remedy, and if all this doesn't work, take an aspirin or ibuprofen.

Spend most of your time in a lighter environment and get outside to exercise at least 20 minutes, every day. Spending time in low-light conditions will make you fatigued and craving carbohydrates (due to vitamin D deficiency), which may trigger headaches. Combining sunlight and exercise will increase your cerebral blood flow, reduce stress hormones and boost serotonin activity in your brain.

Studies suggest that an increased dosage of vitamin B2 riboflavin-rich foods can help prevent migraine headaches. These foods include whole grain products, green leafy vegetables, fruits and non-dairy milk products. Headache symptoms may take up to 4 to 6 weeks to benefit from increasing your riboflavin intake.

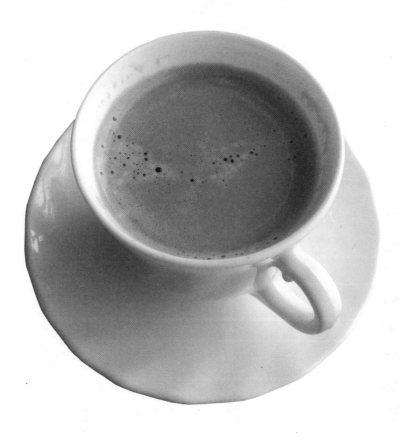

sunday shop, week 3

produce

14 small bananas
large box strawberries
large box blueberries
½ pineapple
1 mango
4+ lemons
½ green cabbage
small bag green beans
1 cucumber
3 tomatoes
1 red onion
1 bunch asparagus
1 bunch cilantro
small ginger root
1 small iceberg lettuce
1 small bag bean sprouts
5 small potatoes
1 portion cherry tomatoes
1 zucchini
2 portions broccoli
1 bunch spinach
1 red bell pepper
1 red jalapeño pepper
1 carrot
1 cob of corn

grocery

1 can organic chickpeas
1 scoop of coconut flakes (if you don't
have any from week 1)

deli

coconut crusted tilapia**
3 oz ahi tuna
2- wild salmon fillets, 3 oz each
3 oz white fish
1 tub non-dairy yogurt
2 liters non-dairy milk

when you get home

Peel bananas, wrap in plastic and store in freezer. Wash produce. Cut tops off strawberries, freeze on baking tray then transfer to storage container. If you can't find precut pineapple halves, get a whole one and use the extra for a sweet treat. You'll only use a quarter this week, so eat the remainder as part of your snack quota.

Buy extra jalapeño pepper and use freely with any dish you want to spice up. **Coconut crusted tilapia is a favorite at *Whistler Fitness Vacations*, but if it's not available in your town, see week 1 shopping list (page 29).

Divide green beans into 4 portions for this week so you aren't left short. You'll have ¾ of the cucumber left over, which you can cut into matchsticks and eat with homemade salsa for a spicy snack.

Stay planet friendly by choosing ahi (yellow-fin) tuna from local waters. Opt for firm white fish (halibut, sole or cod). All fish should be stored in the freezer until the day of usage.

Do you have your fabric bags?

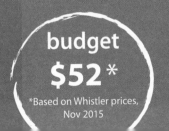

budget
$52*
*Based on Whistler prices,
Nov 2015

day 15

tropical tilapia (fiji)

Set your clock to Fiji time! The unique textures and flavors of the South Pacific can be found at your local market. Invite your friends around for a traditional village feast: sitting on the floor with pillows and mats, feeling like you're worlds away.

1 teaspoon of paprika
pinch chili powder
¼ small onion
1 teaspoon of sesame seeds
3 oz tilapia fillet
¼ head of green cabbage
¼ cucumber
handful of green beans
½ tomato
½ lemon
½ mango

For vegetarian option: Substitute tilapia with sliced firm tofu, sautéed in vegetable broth, spiced with sprinkle of chili peppers and topped with fresh bean sprouts.

Preheat oven to 375°F/180°C.

If you have pre-seasoned fish, then you can just get started. Otherwise, mix ½ finely chopped red jalapeño, ½ cup non-dairy milk, 2 tablespoons crushed gluten-free cereal flakes, 1 tablespoon coconut flakes and 1 tablespoon rice flour in a bowl, then coat fish.

To cook the fish, place it on aluminum foil and bake for 15–20 minutes until middle of the fish is white when you test it with a knife.

Chop cabbage, slice cucumber, trim beans, cut tomato. Peel skin off mango, slice thinly. Pour a few tablespoons of broth into a pan and cook at medium heat until it bubbles. Fry up the spices, add onion and cabbage. Cook until crisp.

Remove fish from the oven, serve with raw cucumber, tomato and mango. Top with sesame seeds and green beans.

calories 444 | carbohydrates 68 g | protein 29 g | fat 10 g
estimated cost $4.45

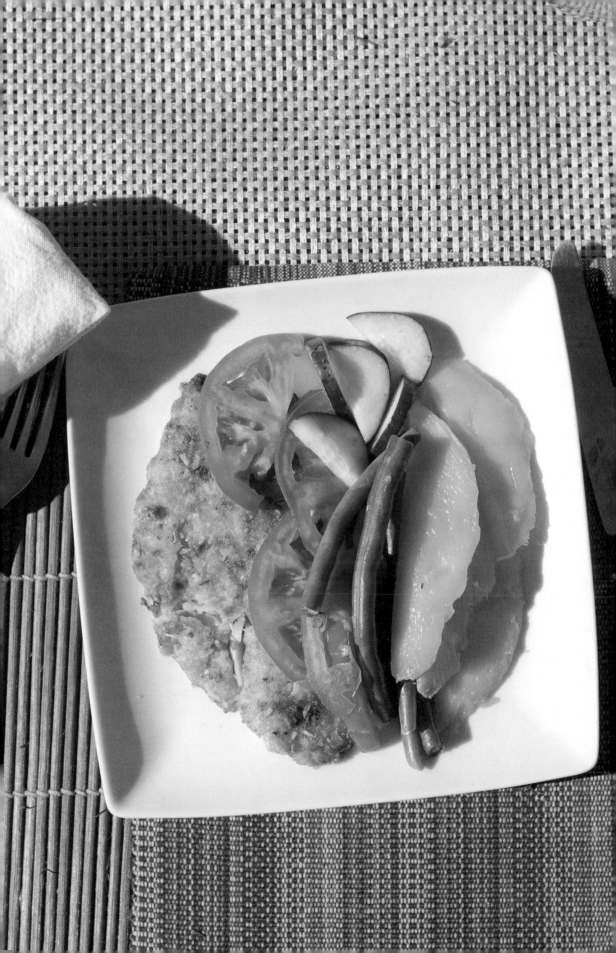

monday

weight:

goals:

notes:

Food	Cost	Time
breakfast		
snack		
lunch		
snack		
dinner		

estimated calories eaten: water:

day 16

sweet and spicy chickpeas (thailand)

The combination of sweet and spicy adds tangy freshness to this scrumptious meal. It's more practical to use the organic canned variety of chickpeas as they are only used once on *The Planet Friendly Diet*... but if you're making a few portions, it's worth cooking from scratch.

1 inch ginger root
1 teaspoon of turmeric
1 teaspoon of paprika
pinch of chili powder
¼ package firm tofu
½ tomato
6 asparagus spears
½ cup cooked chickpeas
handful of green beans
2 leaves iceberg lettuce
¼ cup bean sprouts
¼ cup chopped pineapple
1 tablespoon coconut flakes
½ cup milk alternative

Cut ends off asparagus and green beans. Slice tomato. Remove top and bottom from pineapple, slice off outer skin to remove spikes and holes, cut into thick slices. Place shot glass over middle of each slice and lean into it with your body weight to remove the core.

Smash, peel and chop ginger. Heat a few tablespoons of broth in a pan and cook over medium heat until it begins to bubble.

Fry ginger with turmeric in pan, add tofu and coconut flakes, cook until crisp. Add asparagus, pineapple and green beans; cook until liquid is reduced. Pour milk over vegetables, add chickpeas. Simmer for a few minutes, stirring with wooden spoon.

Serve with lettuce, tomato and bean sprouts.

calories 411 | carbohydrates 68 g | protein 26 g | fat 11 g
estimated cost $3.80

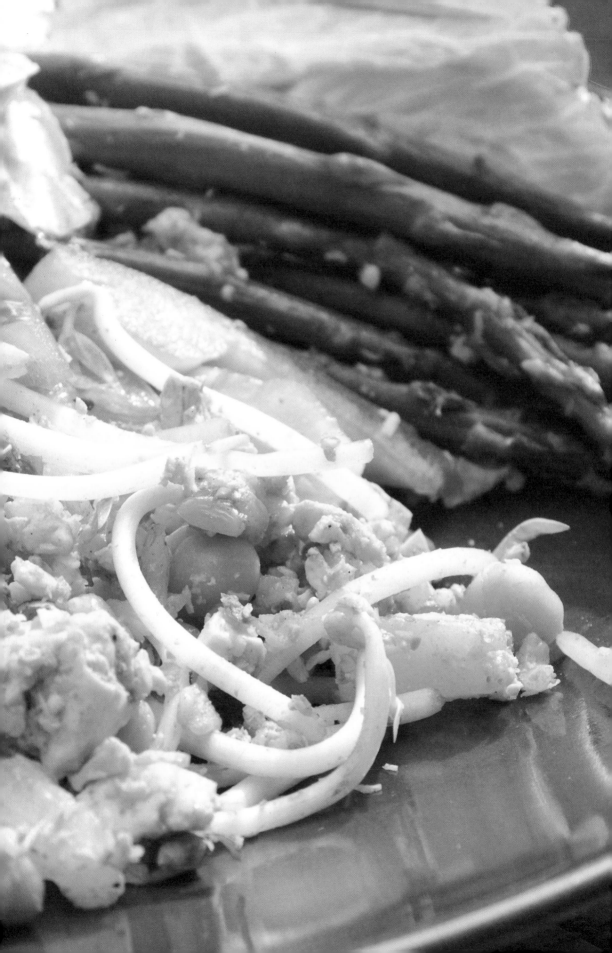

tuesday

weight:

goals:

notes:

Food	Cost	Time
breakfast		
snack		
lunch		
snack		
dinner		

estimated calories eaten: water:

day 17

seared tuna harvest (new zealand)

Fresh tuna steaks are always delicious when seared. You'll get a protein kick from tonight's gourmet meal — it's light but deliciously satisfying. The caramelized crust melts in your mouth, and its meaty flavor makes it a happy substitution for traditional steak!

1 inch ginger root
1 teaspoon of paprika
pinch of chili powder
1 teaspoon of sesame seeds
3 oz ahi tuna
2 sprigs cilantro
5 small potatoes
4–5 broccoli florets
¼ yellow bell pepper
handful of green beans
¼ tomato
1–2 lemons

For vegetarian option: Substitute tuna with tofu skewers (kebab) with pineapple, marinated in a mixture of pineapple juice, garlic, coconut milk and tomato.

Fill bowl with juice squeezed from the lemon and soak tuna in the liquid for 15 minutes. Get the most out of the lemon by sticking a fork in it and twisting until fully juiced. Boil potatoes in a pot of water for 8 minutes, cool and cut into bite-size pieces.

Peel, smash and chop ginger. Chop cilantro finely. Pour a few tablespoons of broth into a pan and cook over medium heat until it bubbles. Add sesame seeds, cilantro, paprika and chili powder — then when tender, add potatoes, broccoli, yellow pepper, green beans and tomato. Simmer 5 minutes, stirring occasionally, adding broth as needed.

Preheat new pan, pour broth in to taste and cook tuna in bubbling liquid for 2 minutes on each side, until lightly crusted. The inside will stay pink, but if it is too undercooked for you, bake at 375°F/180°C for 10 minutes before searing.

Arrange on plate with cooked vegetables. Drizzle lemon juice over tuna, garnish with sesame seeds.

after dinner task:

- make 3 cups of rice with 1 cup dry to 3 cups boiling water (page 23). Refrigerate.

calories 369 | carbohydrates 44 g | protein 30 g | fat 8 g
estimated cost $6.50

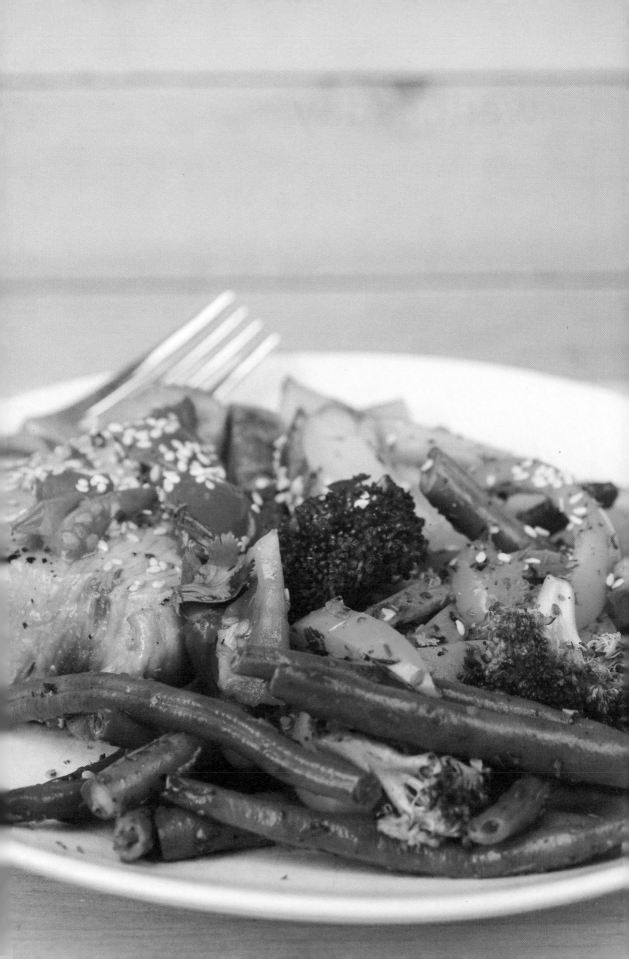

wednesday

weight:

goals:

notes:

Food	Cost	Time
breakfast		
snack		
lunch		
snack		
dinner		

estimated calories eaten: water:

day 18

sock it to me salmon (canada)

Tonight's salmon packs a punch with a spiced-up blend of land and sea, the perfect accompaniment for vibrant green vegetables and fluffy rice. In North America, salmon is in season July to September, although available year-round.

1 clove garlic
1 teaspoon of paprika
pinch of chili powder
2 salmon fillets, 3 oz each
1 lemon
½ zucchini
4–5 broccoli florets
½ cup cooked brown rice
2 tablespoons salsa
pepper

For vegetarian option: Substitute salmon with whole grain quinoa and lightly toasted sesame seeds.

Preheat oven to 350°F/180°C.

Make 2 portions of salsa (page 22). Slice zucchini into thin strips and broccoli into bite-size pieces.

Place salmon on baking tray lined with aluminum foil — 1 for tomorrow. Drizzle lemon juice over fish and bake for 10 minutes. Add zucchini and bake for another 10 minutes. The fish is cooked when, using the tip of the knife, the middle is pink. Wrap tomorrow's salmon (once cooled) and place in the fridge.

Chop garlic finely. Heat a few tablespoons of broth in a pan and cook over medium heat until it bubbles. Fry garlic with paprika and chili powder. Add broccoli and zucchini to the pan, cook until lightly crisp.

Add rice and cook for a few minutes, stirring gently. Serve with salsa and fresh ground pepper.

calories 415 | carbohydrates 62 g | protein 29 g | fat 6 g
estimated cost $4.50

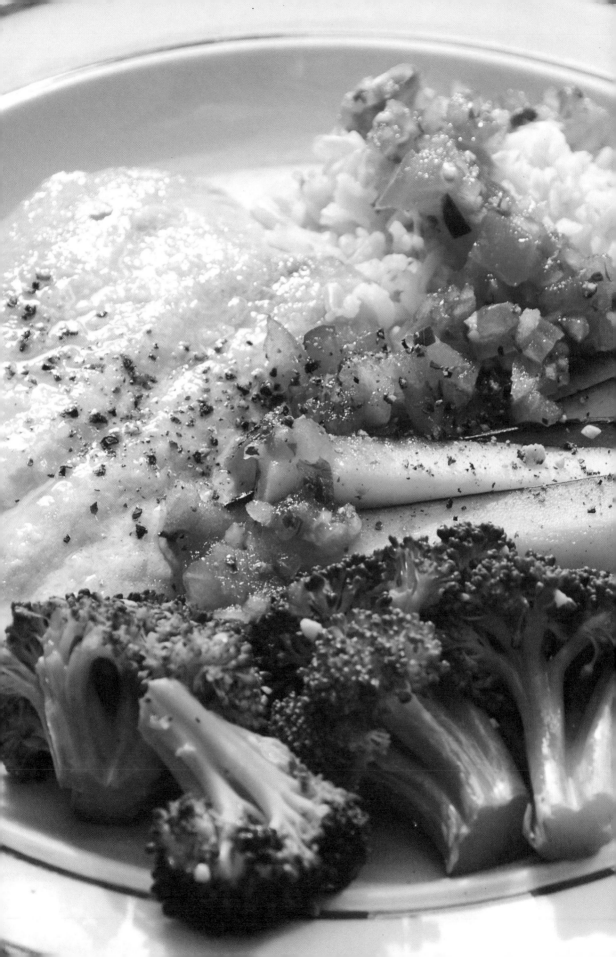

thursday

weight:

goals:

notes:

Food	Cost	Time
breakfast		
snack		
lunch		
snack		
dinner		

estimated calories eaten: water:

day 19

remixed risotto (italy)

Melt-in-the-mouth Italian cuisine is made simple with this nutty salmon mixer. Plan your time to cook the rice — you'll need to keep a close eye on it. Between the tangy lemon, sweet cherry tomatoes and oven-baked salmon, this recipe will make you feel like a genius!

1 clove garlic
1 teaspoon of turmeric
3 oz salmon
handful of spinach
½ zucchini
6 asparagus spears
10 unsalted almonds
5 cherry tomatoes
1 lemon
1 cup cooked brown rice

For vegetarian option: Substitute salmon with 4 chopped mushrooms (sautéed in vegetable broth until soft) and use ½ cup of quinoa instead of brown rice. Simmer ¼ cup of cottage cheese in the pan with cooked mushrooms.

Preheat oven to 350°F/180°C. Slice zucchini and cut ends off asparagus. Juice the lemon. Drench zucchini and asparagus in the juice, place on baking tray and roast for 10 minutes.

While vegetables cook, make the risotto mix: chop garlic finely, pour broth into a large pot and cook over medium heat, cook garlic. Add a few more tablespoons of broth, rice and salmon (break into pieces). Stir gently until liquid is absorbed.

Pile risotto on a bed of raw spinach with asparagus and zucchini. Top with almonds (purchased week 2) and cherry tomatoes.

calories 477 | carbohydrates 60 g | protein 31 g | fat 13 g
estimated cost $4.90

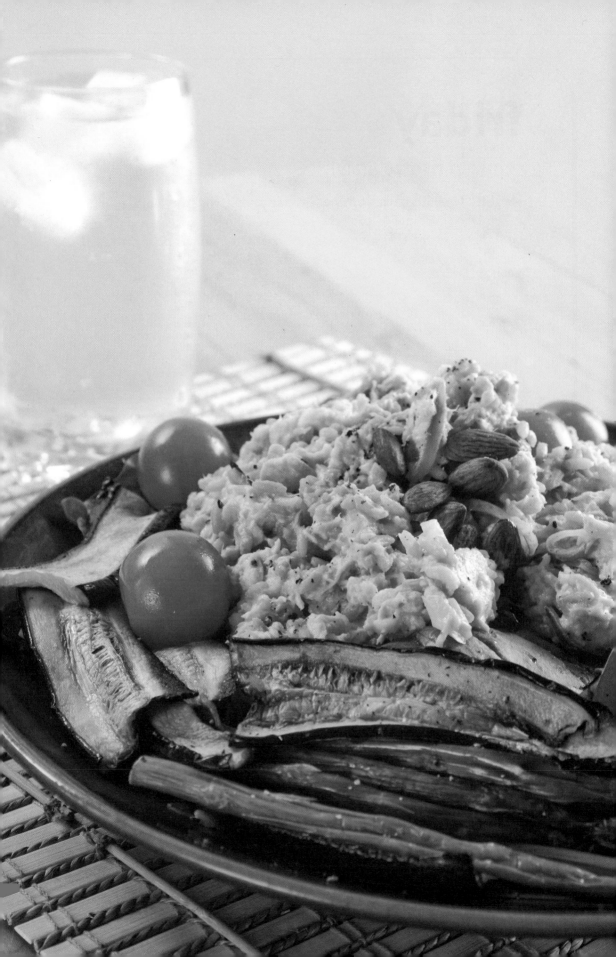

friday

weight:

goals:

notes:

Food	Cost	Time
breakfast		
snack		
lunch		
snack		
dinner		

estimated calories eaten: water:

day 20

kick-ass mango curry (malaysia)

Kick-ass workouts are made possible by kick-ass meals like these! This dish is balanced with a rainbow of vegetables, complemented by the characteristic curry flavors.

1 teaspoon of turmeric
1 teaspoon of paprika
pinch of chili powder
3 oz white fish fillet
6 asparagus spears
1 carrot
½ lemon
½ mango
2 tablespoons coconut flakes
½ cup milk alternative
1 cup cooked brown rice

For vegetarian option: Substitute fish with scrambled tofu and 1 tablespoon of sesame or pumpkin seeds.

Preheat oven to 350°F/180°C. Squeeze lemon over fish and bake 15–20 minutes until center is white when you test with the tip of a knife.

Cut ends off asparagus, slice carrot into thin pieces, peel and chop mango. Heat a few tablespoons of broth in a large pot and cook over medium heat until it bubbles.

Add spices and coconut flakes and fry until lightly brown. Add carrot, asparagus and rice to the pan (rice is in the fridge from day 17). You can also add mango, or keep it uncooked. Pour milk alternative over ingredients and simmer until liquid is reduced. Serve with non-dairy yogurt if desired.

after dinner task:

- defrost black beans and non-dairy cheese by placing in the fridge

calories 395 | carbohydrates 71 g | protein 27 g | fat 7 g
estimated cost $3.85

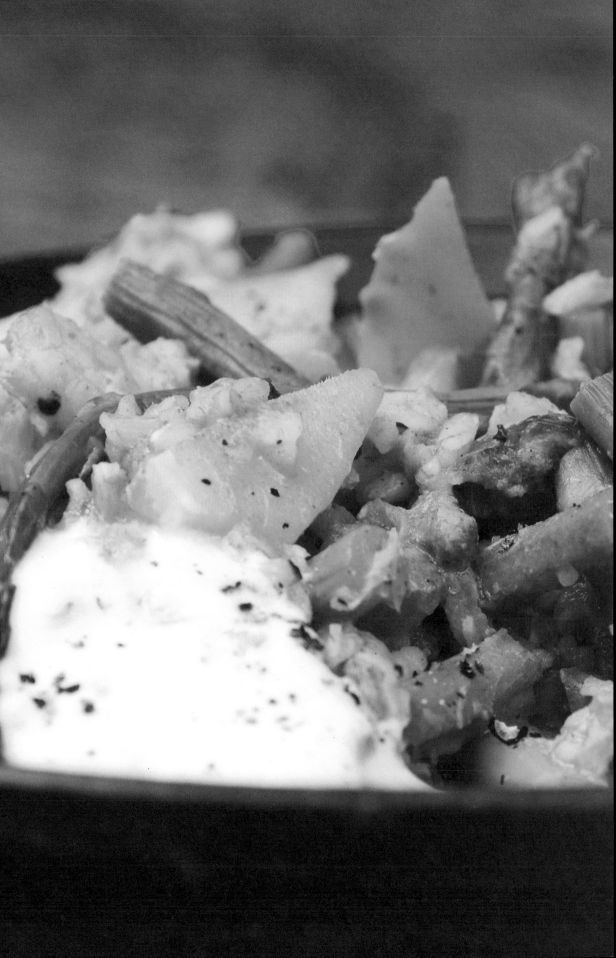

saturday

weight:

goals:

notes:

Food	Cost	Time
breakfast		
snack		
lunch		
snack		
dinner		

estimated calories eaten: water:

day 21

pepper stuffed with awesomeness (mexico)

Greening up your eating patterns is easy with these intensified vegetarian flavors. This contemporary twist on the traditional rice and beans is an exciting way to wrap up 21 days of *The Planet Friendly Diet* challenge. Invite your friends over and celebrate!

1 clove garlic
1 teaspoon of paprika
pinch of chili powder
1 red bell pepper
2 lettuce leaves
½ cup lima beans
1 small cob of corn
½ cup cooked black beans
30 g non-dairy cheese
½ cup cooked brown rice
2 tablespoons salsa

Preheat oven to 350°F/180°C. The rice, black beans and salsa are already made in the fridge. Boil a large pot of water, cook lima beans and corn for 5–7 minutes. Strain in cool running water, pop beans from pods and remove corn kernels by slicing downward.

Remove top and scoop seeds out of red pepper. Chop garlic into fine pieces. Heat a few tablespoons of broth in a large pot and cook over medium heat with garlic and spices. Cook until tender then add corn, lima beans, rice and black beans.

After cooking for a few minutes, transfer ingredients into the pepper. Grate about 2 tablespoons of cheese over top and bake for a few minutes until melted.

Take lettuce leaves and make into a salad bowl by filling with cooked ingredients. Add fresh salsa and enjoy!

calories 431 | carbohydrates 79 g | protein 20 g | fat 8 g
estimated cost $3.60

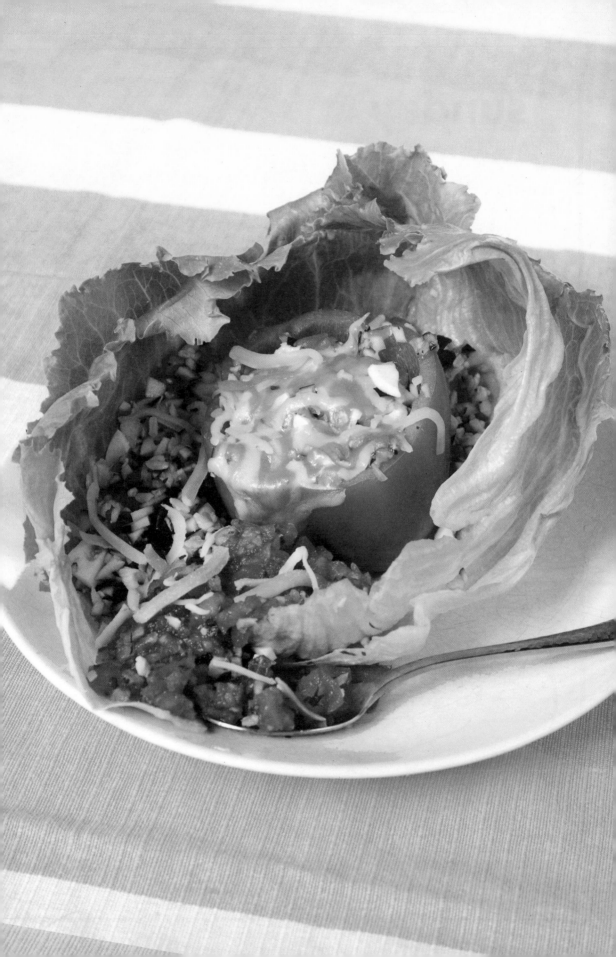

sunday

weight:

goals: ACHIEVED!!!

notes:

Food	Cost	Time
breakfast		
snack		
lunch		
snack		
dinner		

estimated calories eaten: water:

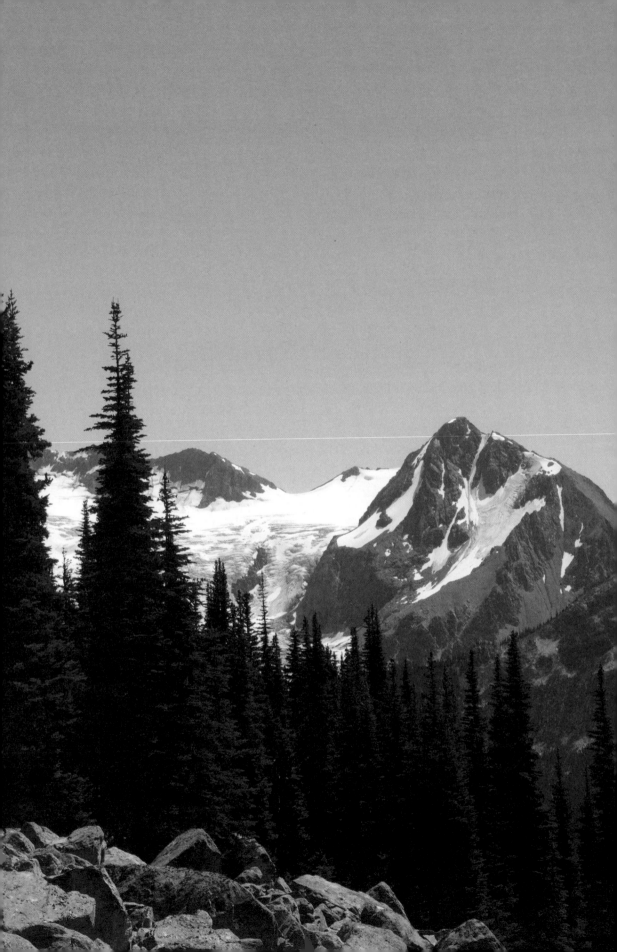

Yay! Congratulations!!

Many people talk about kick-starting their change, but you actually did it! You've successfully completed 21 days! That's awesome. If you came from a background of daily meat eating (like most of my clients), here's breakdown of the impact you had on the world by switching to plant and fish protein for a few weeks:

1. **You Saved Water:** it takes 13,250 liters of water to produce enough crops to feed the cattle that will make just one meat meal. This is about eight times more water than it takes to make a loaf of bread.

2. **Global Warming and Climate Change:** the most damaging greenhouse gas is methane. The primary worldwide source of methane is rearing livestock — this is having a direct impact on global warming and climate change. You helped polar bears keep their home!

3. **Just Like Riding a Bike:** it takes the same amount of greenhouse emissions to drive an SUV for two hours as it does to produce and eat a portion of steak.

4. **Your Choices Helped Feed the Hungry:** by opting for plant or fish protein, the demand for animals decrease. This means that there is more grain left over to feed people, when its not fed to animals. Researchers at Cornell University found that the grain consumed by animals could feed about 800 million starving people.

Now it's time to learn how to make it your own by integrating my principles into your own tastes and preferences. In the next section of this book, you'll learn all the basics of modern nutrition that I use for the nutrition talks at *Whistler Fitness Vacations*. By the end of this book, you'll have all the info needed to never go on a diet again.

—— @icatsmiley ——

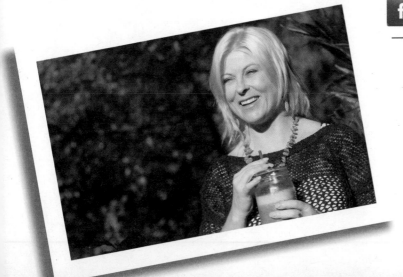

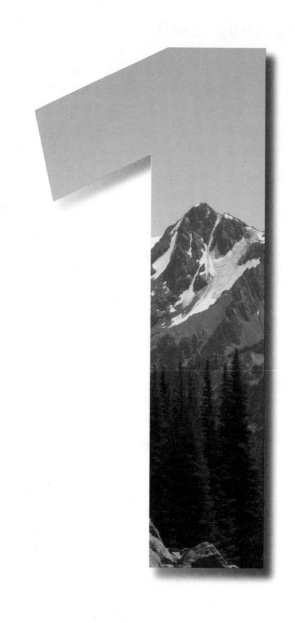

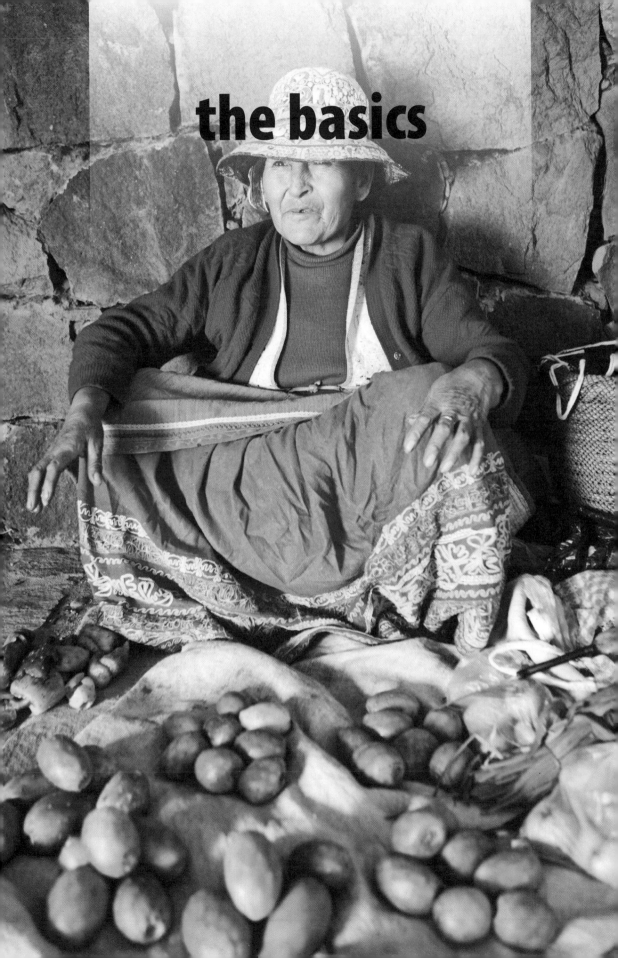

the basics

metabolism

Metabolism is an energy-burning system, like a campfire. The wood keeps the fire going in the same way food keeps you going. If there is too much food in our body to be metabolized, it turns to fat. Put the right amount of wood on the fire, and it will run steadily until you put it out — just like feeding yourself the right amount of food. It's all about energy balance.

Think about all foods that you eat as having a cost, and by the end of the day, you need to have "balanced your account," based on calorie needs. For example, *The Planet Friendly Diet* is about weight loss, so the caloric budget is set at 1,200 calories per day, based on eating every 3 to 4 hours. Did you go for a run today? What else have you eaten today? Will you be blowing your budget tonight at your boyfriend's birthday dinner?

If so, then plan ahead. Bank your calories so that you can "afford" to eat more should the occasion arise. Weight loss is about going into deficit and spending the excess calories that are currently being stored as fat.

did you know....?

Slimming down to your #happysize will help the economy. It doesn't cost more to be a healthy weight, but the consequences of obesity cost everyone a fortune.

- New studies on obesity from *Statistics Canada* suggest that overweight men are nearly four times more likely to be absent from work than co-workers within the healthy weight range.

- If everyone in our community was within healthy weight range, the cost of living could be reduced. Research shows that a company of 1000 employees would save about $285,000 per year if they didn't have to pay out obesity-related health care, and worker sick days. Imagine — this reduced overhead could allow them to drop their prices, saving us money!

- The Canadian Government spends about $5.6 billion per year on diabetes-related care. If people weren't obese, this money could put about $13.2 billion per year back into the economy.
- There's only so much government money to go around, and most of it gets spent on obesity-related diseases. This means that we wouldn't need to do ice bucket challenges and fun runs to raise money for important health research and development simply because there would be enough government money for it.

tip no 8

decide how much food you need

Once you've completed *The Planet Friendly Diet*, you'll need to adapt your caloric needs to suit your body composition goals. Note, the guidelines are based on women's training needs to look their best — not for athletes with performance goals.

To maintain weight but lose fat and gain muscle, on lighter training days eat 300 to 500 fewer calories. Then increase intake for the other days by 300 to 500 calories over 5 small meals. To lose weight by losing fat and gaining muscle, 4 or 5 days per week, eat 1,200 calories like you would normally on *The Planet Friendly Diet*. Then eat 300 to 500 calories more than usual, twice per week on heaviest training days. To bulk up by losing fat and building muscle, 4 or 5 days per week, eat 1,500 to 1,700 calories per day, which means adding 300 to 500 calories to total daily consumption of what you would normally eat on *The Planet Friendly Diet*. Then resume a 1,200-calorie diet 2 days per week — eating 300 to 500 fewer calories than usual. The goal is to put your body into balance so that you can eat 1,700 to 2,000 calories per day while maintaining optimal weight. Eventually you'll be able to eat more and weigh less.

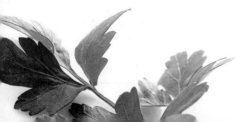

tip nº 9

balance the macronutrients

There are 3 main food groups — carbohydrates, protein and fat (macro-nutrients).

> ## *The Planet Friendly Diet*
> ## three fundamental principals
>
> 1. A meal is when you are eating from all three food groups and it is of 250 calories or more. This will keep hunger away for 2 to 3 hours.
>
> 2. A snack is when you are eating less than 250 calories from 1 or 2 food groups. This will keep hunger away for about an hour.
>
> 3. A mini-meal is when 3 macronutrients are present but you are eating less than 250 calories. This will keep hunger away for about 2 hours.

It takes 20 minutes for the signal of being full to be relayed to the brain. This means that eating slowly, with a knife and fork, and resting the cutlery down between bites will allow enough time for this signal to be processed. This is a very general rule of thumb — everyone's metabolism is different.

If the body does not get all food groups, whatever you eat will be digested as a snack... which means your body will keep looking for its meal by making you feel hungry. For example, an apple and banana is a great pick-me-up because it is a simple carbohydrate (more about that later), but it doesn't have any valuable protein or fat source, so it is good only to tide you over for an hour or two until you eat your next meal. Snacks will always be second best to meals as they are usually low in protein, which is one of the major food groups. The body will crave the macronutrient that it missed the last time you ate, which is why you can sustain your energy for longer if you snack on mini-meals. This is a miniature portion of your meal, with all 3 food groups present, such as an apple and peanut butter. You get carbs from the apple, protein and fat from the peanut butter.

It's important to keep your body charged. Ramp up your snack to include the missing food group — for example, adding some cheese to your rice, beans and fresh salsa will let your body process those calories as a meal, keeping you fuelled for longer.

how much should we eat?

Although calorie counting is not a preferred method of a healthy lifestyle, it's important to be aware that foods contain calories and exercise burns off calories. One pound of body fat is equal to 3,500 calories. This means that if you want to lose one pound of body fat, you must cut 3,500 calories.

Losing body fat can be done by solely reducing food, but it's not a good idea. Severely restricting food can result in depleted fuel stores, muscle wasting, stress fractures, fainting, reduced performance, weakness, fatigue and slowed metabolism. Drastically increasing activity levels is not a viable option either, as intense exercise requires increased nutrition to ensure the body can operate optimally and meet the increased energy needs.

A combination of reduced eating and gradual increased activity will lead to healthy and gradual weight loss.

By eating 250 calories less per day and burning an extra 250 calories by exercise, you'll lose 1 pound per week. That may not seem like a whole lot, but this weight loss, as opposed to others, is more likely to stay off because you've maintained your muscle and kept your metabolism buzzing. Little steps add up! Everybody has a different energy (calorie) requirement. This energy requirement varies based on gender, age, weight, height, type and amount of physical activity. Keep an eye on the scale and boost intake to 1,500 or 1,700 calories as needed to maintain healthy weight and a happy, energized lifestyle.

tip № 10

eat at least 1,500 calories per day

The Planet Friendly Diet is only 1,200 calories, but this is meant as a 60-day program only. Calories matter! The human body needs nutrients to keep us healthy, but we essentially need calories to get the energy needed to live. Calories keep our functions going — digestion, heartbeat, vital organs, brain activity, etc. So dipping too low in calories (below 1,500 – 1,700 calories per day) is detrimental in the long term and will lead to stress on the body, mind and spirit. The important thing about this whole health game is to keep your stride going at a balanced pace and not get obsessed with losing weight and puritanical lifestyles. One of the most trending problems today in holistic health circles is adrenal fatigue syndrome (also known as 21st century stress syndrome, as it is thought to be caused by prolonged stress). Consistently consuming fewer calories than your body needs will lead to some really negative endocrine adaptations; namely, your metabolism and digestion go all over the map, plummeting down with your blood pressure, making you prone to all kinds of things that you don't need in your life, like depression, anxiety, stress, cravings, obsessions, sensitivity to cold, and most of all, working out will be impossible because your body will lose its ability to recover. In other words, your body will respond to being in long-term caloric deficit the same way as anyone suffering from starvation.

Adrenal glands cope with every physical and mental stress that you put them through by releasing a hormone known as cortisol. However, in prolonged stressed conditions, a time comes when adrenal glands get exhausted and are incapable of producing enough cortisol, which is the stage when you are said to be suffering from adrenal fatigue syndrome. Symptoms occur partly due to less hormonal production, which affects all of the body. Examples include continually feeling tired and sleepy, feeling overwhelmed trying to keep up with life's demands, ongoing cravings for sweet and salty snacks, difficulty getting up in the morning even after enough sleep. You may also experience body fatigue, body aches, extreme stress and loss of libido. Several factors are associated with adrenal fatigue syndrome, which may include chronic illness, poor diet, poor lifestyle, chronic stress and therefore less sleep with more physical stress throughout the day. Changing your lifestyle is essential and urgent if you are experiencing any or all of these symptoms. Adrenal fatigue is considered a myth by traditional doctors and researchers as there is no profound basis for this syndrome in medical sciences. Different vitamin supplements and lifestyle changes are prescribed by the adrenal fatigue theory's supporters, but these may be harmful without any genuine need.

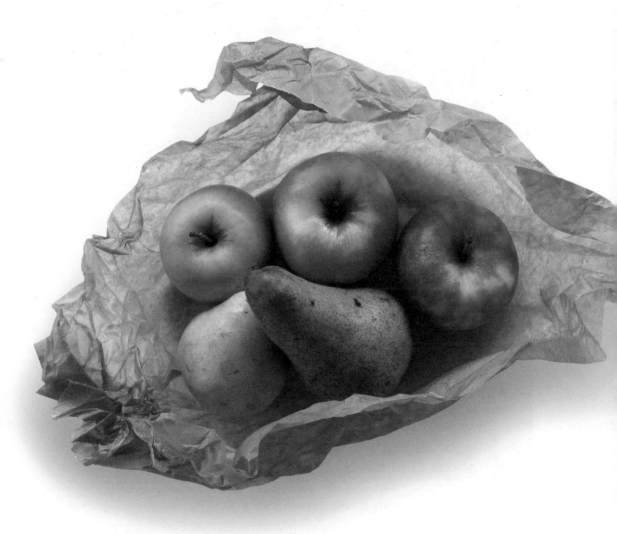

carbohydrates

Carbohydrates are the good guys. They do not make you fat! Many people who go on carb-free diets actually wind up eating more carbs because they don't understand the difference between the two kinds.

simple carbohydrates are like race cars — fast start and sudden stop. They're usually brightly colored, mostly eaten as fruits and vegetables. Easily digested and absorbed into the bloodstream, simple carbs are readily recognized by the body's filing system, which gives an immediate burst of energy followed by a crash. This is when extreme hunger kicks in, usually leading to consumption of whatever is fast and easy.

complex carbohydrates are usually darker colored, such as whole grain products, brown rice, quinoa, lentils, chickpeas and potatoes. They are like a Rolls Royce with a big gas tank, able to cruise at a steady pace for hours. If you break down the molecules in a science lab, you'll find they have a more complicated structure, which means that your body needs a little more time to digest and absorb them into the bloodstream (remember the filing system?). It chips away at metabolizing them over a couple of hours, giving you continual energy while fuelling your body slowly.

Both kinds of carbs are important, but they need to be eaten together to get the full benefit from the fuel being provided.

carbs are sexy

There are lots of weight-loss plans coming out these days that emphasize low carbohydrate intake, and people on these diets are losing a ton of weight in a really short time. That is why many conclude that a very low or almost zero-carb diet is most effective in losing weight — but there's lots more to the big picture that you may not be aware of.

First off, the term "low-carb" is referring to being low in complex carbohydrates, like whole grains (rice, wheat, oats, spelt, quinoa, couscous, barley, bulger) and carbs that are slow burning in our digestive system, but vital to healthy metabolic function — also to brain function and maintaining a balanced personality. Many of my weight-loss clients who have come from low-carb diets before starting my program talk about having problems sleeping, in addition to needing to take laxatives to enable a bowel movement. Complex carbs provide serotonin, which converts to melatonin in our sleep. Without this, it's pretty hard to fall into a deep sleep because the body just doesn't want to. Regarding bowel movement, it's important to keep the gut healthy by having enough insoluble fibers, as this adds bulk to your diet and prevents constipation by removing waste. While insoluble fiber is present in vegetables, whole grains have greater quantities.

Also, complex carbs are essential for our body as they provide instant energy to muscles during aerobic activities. Our body converts excess glucose gained from carbs into glycogen, which is stored in liver and muscle cells for future energy purposes. A normal person contains 400 to 1,000 grams of glycogen. With every 1 part of glycogen, 4 parts of water are also stored, almost 1,600 to 4,000 ml. This means that if you go on a low-carb diet for a while, eventually you're going to have a "cheat day" and crave bread, pasta, mac and cheese, pizza... simply put, your glucose reserves will become exhausted, and your body will tell you that you need to eat carbohydrates now otherwise your body will start consuming your remaining glycogen stores. Not good.

fast weight loss isn't always good

On average, people who jump on a carb-free diet can lose up to 12 lb. of glycogen and stored water in only 4 days of dieting. But it's the depletion of glycogen reserves and the associated water that they are losing, not fat! Once they go back to regular eating, their body will grab the glucose from the bloodstream and will instantly convert it into glycogen to store in the liver and muscles. For each gram of glycogen, the body will take 4 grams of water, and they will gain the whole lost weight back in a single day. This is why people commonly gain weight back after liquid diets, such as cabbage soup, or the renowned detox tonic of lemon juice, maple syrup and cayenne pepper. It was only glycogen and water that they will have lost, as fat is not so quickly oxidized with only this low-carb diet.

The "carbophobic" mentality has led many great people to have really terrible sleeping patterns and even personality disorders. It starts with bad breath and leads to carbohydrate deficit of serotonin being able to be produced naturally in your body, which in turn converts to melatonin in your sleep. Lack of sleep opens a whole other can of worms.

If going low-carb/high-protein, do it for a short period of time. Once you hit goal weight, go back to your regular healthy diet and daily kick-ass workouts. Record your protein, carb and fat intake in an app on your smart phone so that you are on track with the recommended macronutrient ratio in line with your goals.

action steps:

- Keep complex carbohydrate intake to at least 150 grams per day, every day, to ensure that you're getting adequate nutrition. This is still considered low-carb.

- Check your bowel movement; you should have at least two per day. Watch your sleep — if you're not sleeping well, you may be dipping too low in complex carbs.

- Eat a combination of both complex and simple carbs. Complex carbs have more insoluble fiber, while simple carbohydrates balance it with soluble fiber. We need both to stay healthy. Include apples, oranges, pears, cucumbers, nuts, strawberries, celery, green leafy vegetables, grapes, onions, root vegetables.

- Exercise daily. A well-balanced diet and exercise will lead to healthy weight loss without any adverse effects on your body.

- Anytime you eat carbs, try to eat protein and fat with it. Make it a meal. Sometimes it's not about subtracting from your meal, it's about adding the missing macronutrient to make it a mini-meal.

- Eat both complex and simple carbs together, such as adding fresh salsa to your rice and beans. You'll get that quick sugar spike of energy from the natural sugars in the tomato, which will wake up your digestive system and tell it to start metabolising the rice and beans!

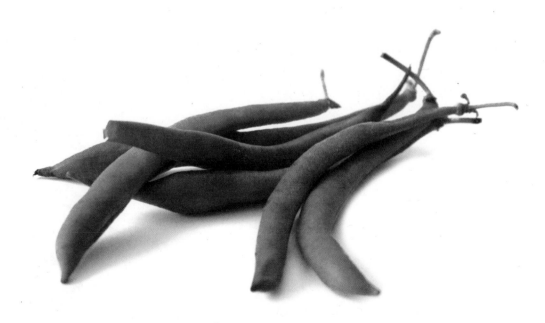

protein

Protein is an important part of having a fast metabolism and looking our best — long and strong nails, shiny hair, beautiful skin and great muscle tone.

Plants (soy, almonds, oatmeal) and animals (tuna, chicken breast, salmon) are sources of protein. Protein provides 4 calories, per gram of energy, to the body, which means that it is not a great source of energy; however, it takes longer to break down in our digestive system, which keeps us fuller for longer. Proteins are a top priority and best eaten in combination with the other food groups: fats and carbs.

You can find quality sources of protein from soy, almonds, oatmeal, tofu, pulses, grains and other food. Protein, minerals and vitamins are the building materials for a healthy structure essential for strong bodies. Protein is what builds your cells: your hair, fingernails, skin and muscle.

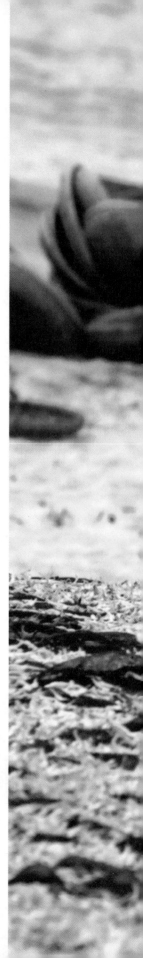

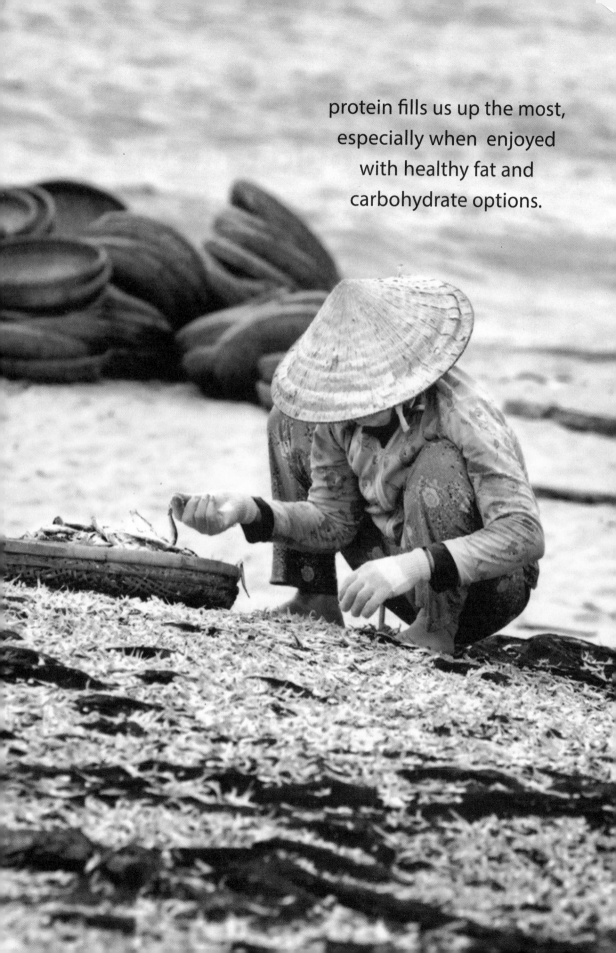

protein fills us up the most,
especially when enjoyed
with healthy fat and
carbohydrate options.

tip no 13

protein should take up a third of your plate

Excess protein results in weight gain and unnecessary strain on your kidneys. On the flip side, lack of protein results in the body breaking down precious muscle mass, which can provide extremely disappointing results for those training and trying to lose weight. Either way, too much or too little protein intake is detrimental.

Women with the goal of being slim should strive for 15 to 25 grams of high-quality protein in every meal. This is based on having protein intake between 10 and 35% of total daily energy — about 0.8 g of protein, per kg of body weight, per day. Find the exact number by multiplying your weight (in kilograms) by 0.8 g. One kilogram is 2.2 pounds. Those with more muscle mass, calculate your weight by 1 to 1.4 grams. An average 3 oz fish portion (100 g) has about 20 g of protein.

Counterbalance the adverse effects of high protein intake with large amounts of calcium from green leafy vegetables, in addition to lots of vitamin C and healthy nutrients from fresh fruit, to maintain adequate dietary fiber levels.

 The Planet Friendly Diet was really easy to follow, I'm not much of a cook but the recipes in it were simple to make — I learnt how to incorporate my regular diet to follow the principals of the book. I lost about 30 pounds the first 8 weeks I was following this book, and now my total weight loss a year later is around 55 pounds.

— Laurisa Stebeleski, Pemberton, Canada

tip nº 14

become a legume lover

Legumes include all lentils, beans, peanuts and peas. Pulses are the edible seeds that grow on these legumes. Generally they refer to the same group of foods — both are an awesome gluten-free, high-protein, high-fiber carbohydrate. Canada is one of the world's largest growers and exporters, with more than 90% of legumes sent to the Middle East, Turkey, India, North Africa, South America and Europe each year.

These healthy foods are rich in protein, fiber, B vitamins, minerals and disease-fighting phytochemicals. At the time of writing, there are almost 50 over-the-counter drugs used to reduce gas in the digestive tract for people who have bloating and flatulence caused by legumes. What users do not realize is that these discomforts only happen when you don't combine amino acids. For most people, the only legumes that can be eaten without plant-protein combining are raw green beans, bean sprouts, alfalfa and green peas. Aim to include 3 cups of legumes per week in your diet, including sources such as black peas, chickpeas, kidney beans, soybeans and tempeh, lima beans, adzuki beans, tofu, miso, mung pea, fava beans, peanuts.

Some people with nut allergies can still eat peanuts because it is a legume, not a nut. Legumes come from a family of plants (*leguminosae*) that have multiple seeds attached to their pods, and although the peanut is inside a hard shell, the seed is not attached to its inside wall.

> protein keeps you feeling fuller for longer because it takes longer to digest.

tip nº 15

amino amigos

You should include more grains, legumes, veggies, nuts and seeds into your diet on a daily basis. If you pass gas so much or get bloated when you eat beans, it's not about Pepto-Bismol; it's about getting all your amino acids. Remember that next time you head to Mexico:)

You see, protein makes its way into the body as tiny little building blocks called amino acid. Out of the 20 known amino acids, we need to get 9 from our diet. These are called essential amino acids because you have to find them from your diet to make sure that your tissues can replenish themselves.

High-quality, complete protein is defined by all essential and non-essential amino acids being present in the food. Plant-protein combining is a theory that makes it really simple to get all amino acids together in one dish, which will create the protein source that is used most efficiently to promote body maintenance and growth. You don't have to eat like this at every meal; as long as you're eating a variety of healthy foods from all groups every day, you'll get enough high-quality protein to optimize your digestion and metabolism.

Successful plant-protein combining is a vegetarian theory that was made popular in 1971 in Frances Moore Lappé's bestseller, *Diet for a Small Planet*. Nutrition experts and medical professionals now agree that this principle is outdated to follow for every meal; however, it remains useful to spread your protein combination sources throughout the day when making your dietary choices.

action steps

- Add chickpeas to any salad for a high-fiber boost. Especially good with baby greens, cilantro, finely chopped tomato and home-made sesame dressing.
- Top tofu and vegetable stir-fry (legumes and veggies) with sesame seeds. In fact, top anything with sesame seeds.
- You've made some quinoa with raisins and slivered almonds along with some spices. Add some zucchini, red pepper, or grated carrot into the mix, and you're dishing up another complete protein meal.

excess protein results in weight gain and an unnecessary strain on your kidneys.

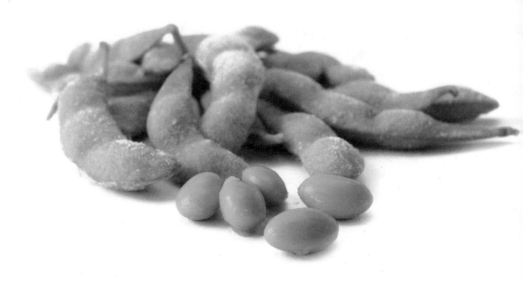

tip nº 16

plan your protein

Protein fills you up because it takes longer to digest. It's important to find the right balance — eating too much will put strain on your kidneys and (like eating too much of anything) make you fat.

Low-protein diets are not recommended as they will cause you to lose valuable muscle mass, which makes it harder to recover from your workouts. They will also lower your metabolism as you'll have less muscle mass. If you've ever wondered why a man can eat more than a woman of roughly the same size and not gain weight, it could be because of his muscle mass.

Time management and organization is super important when it comes to cooking balanced meals.

action step

- If you're on the run, whip up a Super Smoothie — my amazing recipe of frozen berries, banana, non-dairy milk, orange juice, spinach, protein powder and non-dairy yogurt blended on high for 10 seconds. This is my best tip for staying on track for those crazy busy days when you don't feel like the "eating experience," you just need the meal.

fat

Fat is an important part of a healthy diet and is most easily digested when eaten with protein and carbohydrate. Like carbs, fat feeds the brain and balances emotions. It protects the kidneys, liver and heart, helping to regulate body temperature. Fat is the easiest food group to overeat, as the rate of absorption is slower, which means it takes longer for you to feel full. Plus, there are more than twice as many calories per gram of fat compared to carb or protein sources.

Fat and oil consumption should consist mainly of unsaturated fats, vegetable oils and soft margarines that are low in trans and saturated fats. Limit saturated fats such as lard, butter, shortening and hard margarine.

Most taste buds enjoy the creamier, richer and smoother foods, but you will greatly benefit in your weight-loss journey and overall health by using only a little taste of fat. When we take a hard look at our dietary patterns, it's humbling to realize how many low-quality food sources we are eating every day, contributing to the consumption of way too many calories.

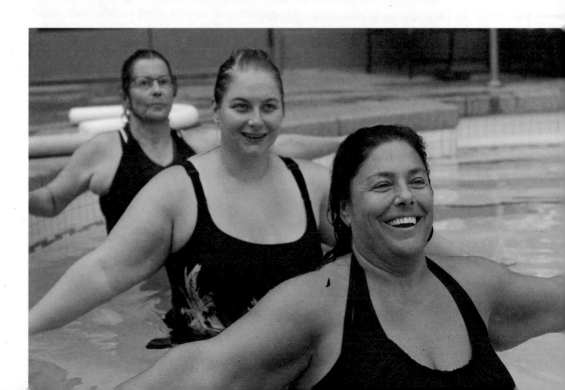

tip nº 17

fat doesn't make you fat

good fat Unsaturated fat is the healthy kind, found in foods like nuts, avocados, fish, olive oil and seeds. However, nuts are easy to overeat and, like any fat source, are high in calories, so be cautious of your portion size; 1 serving is about 10 nuts. Seeds are a good alternative to nuts, and they are higher in protein — with sunflower seeds having the highest protein content of all. Get into the habit of scattering sunflower, sesame or melon seeds into salads or soups, using seeds as toppings for bread or stirring them into your cooking. It helps you achieve your fat and protein daily requirements, making the food tastier at the same time, especially for vegetarians.

bad fat Foods high in saturated fats, such as butter, cheese, whole milk, egg yolk, sausage, hamburger and bacon, should be avoided or used sparingly. If a fat source looks solid at room temperature, it is saturated, which means you should allow yourself no more than 1 serving per day. As a society, we eat way too much saturated fat, and as saturated fat is high in cholesterol, it clogs up our arteries, which can eventually lead to heart disease, stroke and excess body fat.

fat is the easiest food group to overeat as the rate of absorption is slower, which means it takes longer for you to feel full.

Choose "real" foods first, for example, use butter first and non-hydrogenated margarine second. Fat and oil consumption should consist mainly of unsaturated fats, vegetable oils and soft margarines that are low in trans and saturated fats.

Oil and fat consumption should not exceed 2 to 3 tablespoons per day. That little amount is a whopping 220 to 330 calories!

action step

- Fat-free America has never been more obese, partly because fat alternatives just keep you hungry for more. While they are usually half the calories, we eat twice as much. As a golden rule, treat treats like the treats that they are — enjoy your full-fat ice cream occasionally and be satisfied and happy with just 1 portion.

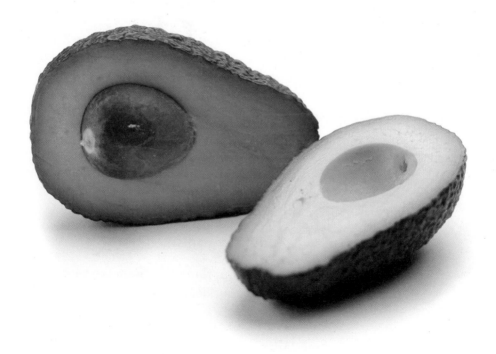

portion sizes

Always check the nutrition label for portion sizes so you know how much fuel is going into your body. You don't always have to have one portion of things, but try always to be aware of how many portions you are about to eat, so that you can balance out the other macronutrients (page 130).

Your hand clenched as a fist, or a baseball, represents:

- 1 medium fruit (1 serving)
- 2 servings of grain (1 cup)

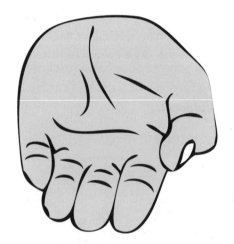

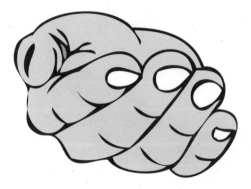

Your entire thumb or 2 dice together represents:

- 1 serving of cheese (1 ounce/ 30 grams)

Your thumb tip, from the second knuckle, represents:

- 1 serving of added fat or oil (1 teaspoon)

The palm of your hand (excluding fingers), or a deck of cards, represents:

• 1 serving of meat/fish

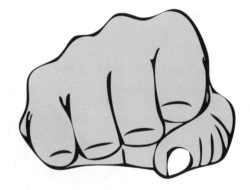

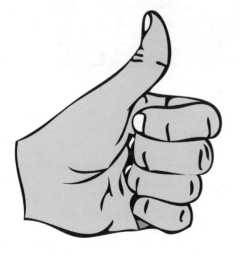

1 hand cupped, side up, represents:

• 1 serving of grain (½ cup)

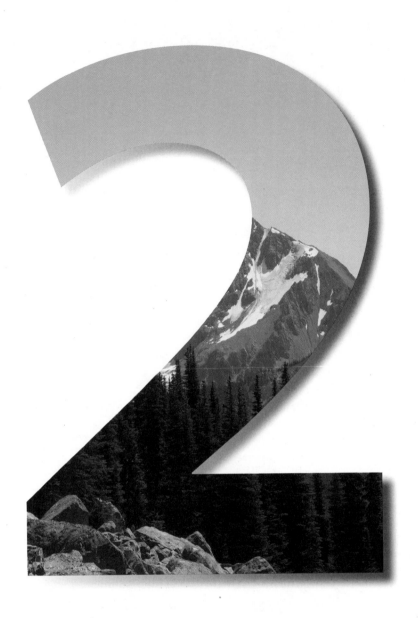

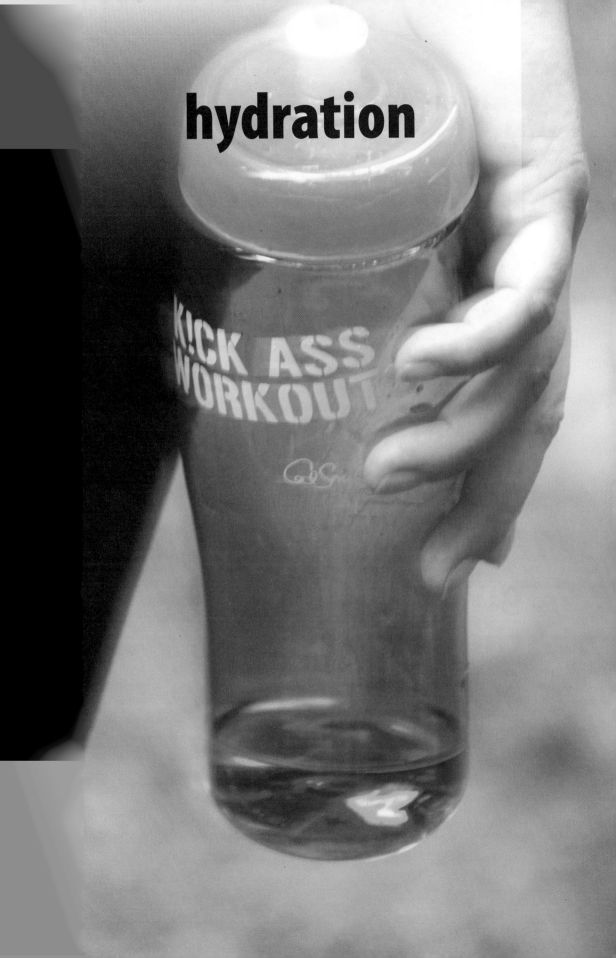

hydration

water

Everything in your body needs water to function properly, including breathing, digestion, metabolism, waste removal and temperature regulation. Water controls many different reactions in your body and is responsible for transportation of nutrients via the blood such as oxygen. And this we can't live without!

People who are overweight, tired or stressed usually have not had enough water. Dehydrated, they can feel tired, sluggish and irritable. Thirsty people often develop extreme cravings for food, misreading the signals their body is sending them to drink water.

Staying hydrated throughout the day is vital for every aspect of your health, from your fat-burning ability to attention span. Check your hydration levels by keeping an eye on your urine when you go to the bathroom. It should be clear. If it's not, get drinking!

tip no 18

give bloating the boot

Maximize your water absorption and reduce bloating by reducing sodium and increasing potassium intake (eat more bananas, apricots, spinach and salmon). It's much better to have the water you drink actually move through your body, instead of just sitting there!

tip no 19

carry a water bottle everywhere

Make drinking part of your routine by taking a reusable water bottle everywhere with you. Keep track of how many times you refill it to meet your 4-liter goal.

tip no 20

drink all day

Drink 4 liters of water a day when you are exercising — 2 liters before noon and 2 more liters before 5 pm. On the days that you're not exercising, drink 3 liters. It seems like a lot of water at first, but once you get used to it, you'll quickly see a boost in your energy levels and muscle recovery. Although water is not the only way to hydrate, it's the best way. You'll boost your health in so many ways and look much better too: clearer skin, shinier hair, fewer wrinkles!

There's been debate over whether other liquids (like coffee, tea, milk, juice and soda) count towards your daily liquid total. In the end, most nutritional authorities believe that they should be included. However, in the case of good, better, best, there is no beverage that will benefit your body more than natural spring water.

Many people in the world have to walk miles to find clean drinking water, and yet so many people neglect to hydrate themselves on a daily basis. We have an amazing natural resource, right in our kitchen — drink up!

Water keeps our cells and body systems running smoothly. It is used to maintain blood volume, which is imperative for regulating body temperature and delivering oxygen and nutrients to the rest of the body. Every cell of your body needs water to function properly.

tip nº 21

caffeinate your workouts

Try to stay under 300 mg of caffeine per day, without sugar, as long as you're meeting the recommended water intake. Plan your caffeine cycle by learning these numbers: each 1 oz shot of espresso has about 75 mg of caffeine, 8 oz of brewed black coffee has 140 mg, 8 oz of black tea has 45 mg. For example, you can have 4 shots of espresso per day — or 2 shots of espresso and one brewed cup.

Caffeine can boost athletic performance. Researchers have found that caffeine releases calcium, enabling athletes to run with better performance. Caffeine tricks your muscles into releasing more of the calcium needed to contract and relax, making muscle contraction stronger. The brain's perception of feeling pain and fatigue is delayed, which means that you can push yourself physically for longer.

Green bean coffee extracts are an effective and inexpensive way to reduce body weight and prevent obesity in overweight people, and as it is a herbal product, it's safe and doesn't have any adverse effects compared to other chemical weight-loss products on the market. An epidemiological study on mice showed that green bean coffee extracts inhibited fat absorption, and the chlorogenic acid was involved in decreasing the level of triglycerides in the liver, hence reducing weight gain.

action steps

- Coffee is an "anti-nutrient" that can get in the way of normal vitamin and mineral absorption, including iron, magnesium, zinc and potassium. Coffee drinkers, should drink more water than non-coffee drinkers, and unless you pay special attention to your calcium intake, caffeine can leach calcium out of your bones, which will make them more brittle.

- If coffee is the first thing you put into your system in the morning, add a hundred calories or so of carbohydrate to minimize the acidic effect. Try a non-dairy latte or a slice of whole wheat toast if drinking your coffee black.

- Learn to love black coffee. Savour the taste of the bean — a large mocha with whip, or a caramel frappe is full of saturated fat and calories.

- Stay away from coffee if it gives you heartburn or makes you feel nauseous — opt for tea instead. Tea, which also contains caffeine unless it is herbal or caffeine-free, is full of antioxidants and fat-burning qualities!

tip nº 22

drink less alcohol

Alcohol is an anti-nutrient that strips your body of valuable nutrients eaten during the day. If you booze it up too much, your body will start craving high-fat, greasy foods as a way to recover from the nutrient depletions, as your body is out of balance and it is looking for the easiest food to replenish itself. This is because fat makes your body take longer to realize it is full, and there are more than twice as many energy calories per gram of fat as there are per gram of protein and carbohydrate; therefore, fat is the easy choice for your digestive system.

On the upside, drinking small to moderate amounts of alcohol (less than 6 servings per week) is related to lowered blood pressure, which improves blood flow and oxygen delivery to the body tissues.

Serving sizes vary based on the drink; for example, a serving of red or white wine is 5 ounces. Many restaurants serve bigger pours than the recommended serving size, and the size of the wine goblets can make a 5-ounce serving look very small. Try white wine spritzers — mix equal parts wine with soda water and serve with a lemon or lime twist. It's refreshing and stretches the drink out longer.

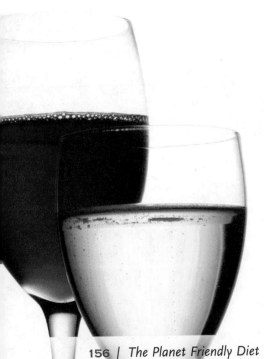

action step

After a night of drinking, you'll feel dehydrated and depleted of vitamins. The best hangover food is high in vitamin C and protein, such as scrambled egg whites with spinach and a slice or two of cheese on toast, with tomato. Drink coffee, then start drinking 2 liters of water. It will take you about 3 hours to drink 2 liters of water, but it'll get you ready to move on with your day.

tip no 23

avoid alcohol when injured

Alcohol can slow down your healing process. The beverage in question is a known vasodilator that opens the arteries, increasing blood flow (which is exactly what you are trying to achieve from your workouts), yet when inflammation becomes part of the equation, alcohol is your worst enemy, especially during the first couple of days after an injury.

Acute inflammation is the body's initial response to harmful stimuli and is achieved by increased activity of plasma and leukocytes from the blood and injured tissues. Chronic inflammation eventually leads to a progressive shift in the type of cells located at the injured site, with simultaneous healing and destruction of tissue due to the inflammation process.

Within the first 72 hours of injury, stay away from alcohol, due to its ability to increase blood flow, numb the brain and alter your pain perception. Masking the pain also masks the ability to protect yourself from further injury, increasing the likelihood of causing more damage.

know how to party

Between catching up with friends and family, fabulous soirées and, of course, those festive celebrations, some weeks are all about eating, drinking and being merry! If you stay on track most of the time, a little bit of indulgence and carefree eating can be loads of fun. So kick back and enjoy this time, minimize weight gain and look forward to getting back on track after the celebrations.

action steps

- If there's a party close to home, why not throw on your warmest winter jacket and power walk there instead of getting a designated driver. Carry your dress shoes, grab your friends and burn off the extra calories you'll be eating at the event!

- Don't arrive hungry. Many diet-conscious people blow their calorie budget on the buffet dinner, skipping breakfast and lunch the next day. This confuses the body and slows down your metabolism — otherwise known as "yo-yo dieting." Consistency is your best bet, mini-meals throughout the day keep you energized, reducing temptation to overeat at night.

- Pick your battles — when every appetizer tantalizes your taste buds, it's easy to forget how hard you worked this year to keep your weight down. Remember the days you really didn't want to go to the gym, but you went anyway.

- Taste new things but keep portion sizes small. Mystery recipes often have mystery fat calories. Keep your hands busy (drink in one hand, purse in the other) and conversation flowing to avoid the host continually offering you more. The drink doesn't have to be alcoholic — and if you're trying new drinks, pace yourself.

- Have a kick-ass workout before you go. Even 20 minutes is better than nothing. Get outside every-day — the fresh air is priceless. Happy living is about sustaining mental, physical and social well-being.

- Relax your calorie counting. Sometimes getting offtrack can refresh your enthusiasm for healthy living. The important thing is to stay healthy enough to be physically ready to get back into it.

tip no 25

coca-cola is not it

Diet soda drinkers often have the school of thought that they are "saving on calories," therefore justify eating more food in their daily total. Regular Coca-Cola has about 10 teaspoons of sugar, but keep in mind that Coca-Cola uses high-fructose corn syrup in their soft drinks due to relatively high sugar prices in the U.S. Save sodas and juices as treats — once in a while as part of a balanced diet. New studies show that the BPA of pop cans may cause premature puberty. So if you feed your kids pop, they'll lose their childhood sooner. That's not cool.

The reason we like Coca-Cola so much is pretty similar to the reason that junkies like heroin. It works the same way on our pleasure sensors. Within 20 minutes of drinking soda, blood sugar spikes causing insulin burst and your liver to turn any sugar into fat. Within 40 minutes, pupils dilate, blood pressure rises, and the adenosine receptors in your brain are blocked, which caused drowsiness despite all caffeine absorption being complete. Within 45 minutes, your body ups the dopamine production, which stimulates the pleasure centers of your brain... tricking you into thinking that it was an enjoyable experience.

Even if you are eating fruits and vegetables, the sodium found in soda will strip your body of these nutrients, namely potassium. Soda will contribute to asthma, kidney issues, obesity, heart disease and eczema. Every time you drink a soda, your risk of obesity increases 1.6 times. People who drink soda are more likely to be smaller in their bone structure because soda breaks down bones with its high concentration of phosphoric acid, which means that when you urinate, you'll pee out all the good calcium you've been eating in your diet, which will deprive your bones of this important mineral.

Diet soft drinks are a good first step for people who come from a highly toxic way of eating and are trying to reduce sugar intake; however, they are not a healthy choice on a regular basis. Artificial sweeteners make you crave real sugars — and although fruit juice is better for you than diet pop, it's still loaded with sugar.

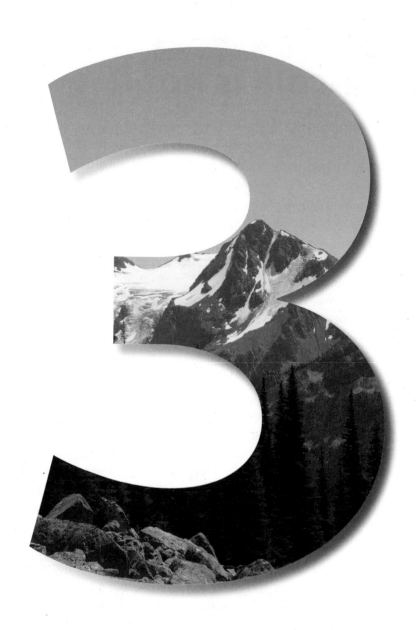

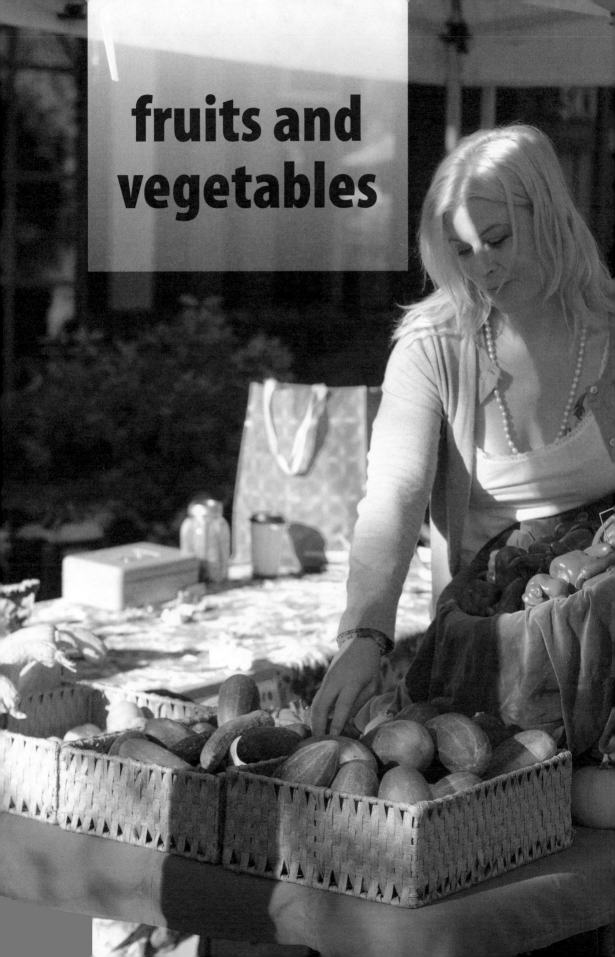

fruits and vegetables

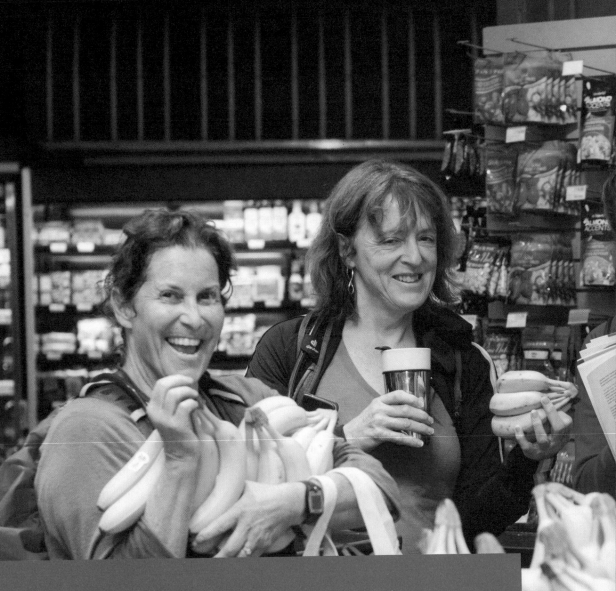

whole food

The whole food revolution has had a big influence on our eating patterns over the past few years. More people than ever before are jumping on board with using vegetables in recipes — not just accompaniments, or side dishes. Make them into soups, toss them in stir-fry, spice them into hot pots or thread them onto kebab skewers. Possibilities are only limited by your imagination!

Low in calories and high in water content, fruits and veggies are super-foods, able to cure illness and prevent deadly disease. Modern medicine is no match for the green prescription, with vegetables being so versatile in any dish and fruit being straight-up nature's candy; there's something for everyone's taste.

Produce is power-packed with fiber and loads of disease-fighting antioxidants. There are so many types to choose from, and if you don't like one type of fruit or vegetable, simply find another. Just resist the temptation to load on the butter and salt — learn to love their natural taste.

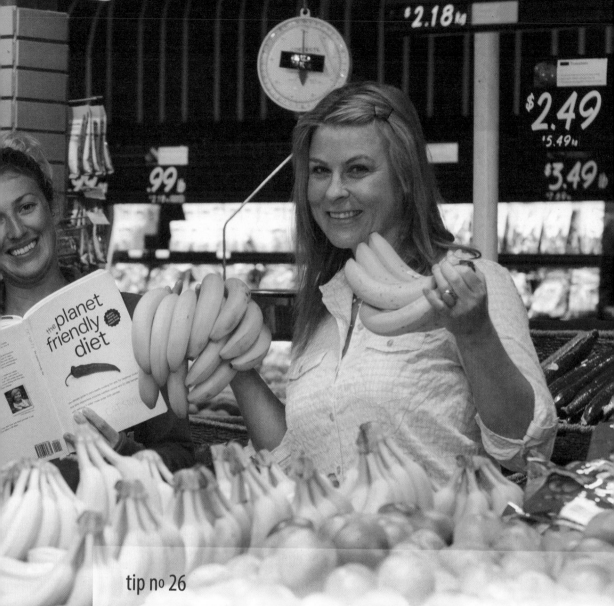

tip № 26

get passionate about produce

Fresh organic produce should be top priority in our food choices — women between 19 and 50 should eat 7 or 8 servings of fruit and vegetables, while men within the same age range should eat up to 10 servings per day.

Just to get an idea of how simple it is, let's walk through a sample day. In the morning, stir ½ cup of blueberries into your yogurt (1 serving). Before working out, grab a banana (1 serving). With lunch, you have a small salad to start (2 servings) and a cup of tomato soup (1 serving). With dinner, have half an ear of corn (1 serving) and a side of steamed spinach (1 serving). For dessert, have a bowl of fresh strawberries (1 serving).

tip №27

buy organic local produce

Happy people, happy food — shopping local not only feels better, it also makes a valuable contribution to your community through economic growth and well-being. *The Planet Friendly Diet* includes all of the most soul-nurturing produce, with most items grown in North America. Yet like everything, balance is key — it's not always viable to shop local. People in volcanic countries might have pineapple and banana available to them, but need to buy imported apples, for example. For them, apples may be the "treat" that pineapple is to North Americans (except in Mexico of course). We also source our complex carbs most commonly from grains — rice and breads — whereas this might be considered a luxury item in Polynesian countries that don't cultivate rice or wheat and aren't on the export route for countries that do. For them, starchy root vegetables like potatoes, kumara and yams provide their main carb source. On a nutritional level, one of the key goals is to fuel your body with vitamin C and magnesium, so it doesn't really matter what fruit and vegetable you eat, as long as it's got the vitamins and minerals needed to convert the amino acids eaten into serotonin and dopamine. These are the neurotransmitters in our brain that trigger pleasure and positivity — making you feel happy!

For years, countries around the world where dairy is not indigenous sourced their calcium and iron from an abundance of green leafy vegetables — grown in their backyard, which you may have the opportunity to do if you have the climate and space. Plant some cabbage, kale, spinach and collard to start, then tomatoes and herbs. Gardening may become your passion — growing your own food can be a powerful kick towards a more organic, wholesome lifestyle.

> by supporting local farmers and grocers, you help boost the local economy.

Living near the sea means epic fish markets! If you're lucky enough to live on the coast, make wandering down to the wharf a weekly ritual — selecting your catch-of-the-day from the fish market, fresh off the boat. Wild fish from the ocean live off a natural diet, which is partly why seafood provides such a concentrated source of essential fatty acids. These can be just as mood elevating as the perfect plant-protein combinations.

Weekend farmers' markets are common in most areas and a great place to pick up fresh in-season produce, while supporting local business at the same time. For products you can't source locally, buy fair trade. This ensures that the farmer is paid fairly, which means their employees are more likely to be treated fairly, contributing to the planet friendly goal of this diet.

Natural foods are always best. The *American Academy of Environmental Medicine* recently stated that genetically modified foods pose a serious health risk in the areas of toxicology; allergy and immune function; reproductive health; metabolic, physiologic and genetic health.

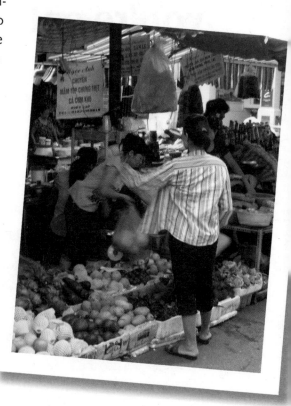

tip nº 28

learn how to make salad dressing

Most dressings are a mixture of fat, acid and flavorings that act as carriers for the fat-soluble vitamins in the raw salad vegetables.

Good dressings should blend well with your salad, bringing out the natural flavors of the ingredients. Choose good olive or nutty sunflower oil and add fresh lemon juice or vinegar for an acidic zest.

Mix 3 parts oil with 1 part acid, add lots of fresh ground pepper and whisk with a fork. Add fresh parsley or basil to taste.

tip nº 29

understand what you're eating

Ingredients for the recipes in *The Planet Friendly Diet* were carefully selected based on their taste and thermogenic and nutritional properties. Learn
about their super powers and integrate them into your independent meal
choices.

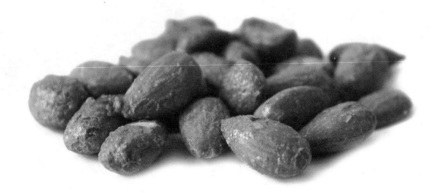

almonds are high in monounsaturated fats (the healthy kind) and can
help reduce the risk of heart disease while lowering cholesterol. They are
bursting in antioxidants and make a great snack (10 is a portion). Get
them in the bulk food aisle and store in an airtight container.

asparagus is packed with nutrients with a juicy taste and delicate flavor. It is affordable at most supermarkets in season. Choose slender firm stems with purple or deep green tips. Store in the fridge the day of purchasing — wrap the ends in a damp paper towel, place in a plastic bag away from light. Use within 2 days — cook the leftover stalks in boiling water for a few minutes, cool, cover with plastic wrap and freeze.

avocado Because up to 90% of its calories are fat, portion size is limited to one-eighth. Cut into 8 pieces when you come home from the market, squeeze a lemon over them, cover individually with plastic wrap and freeze. Thaw a portion overnight in the fridge when you need it. One person won't get through 8 servings of avocado over the next 3 weeks, so mash up the remainder with egg yolk and apply to your hair for 15 minutes as a deep-conditioning hair mask.

bananas are a potassium powerhouse, awesome for regulating water balance and accelerating workout recovery. They help reduce headaches when trying to break habits, like smoking and sugar. Keep a couple of days worth of bananas fresh in the fruit bowl, and store the others in the freezer — peel the skin off and plastic wrap individually.

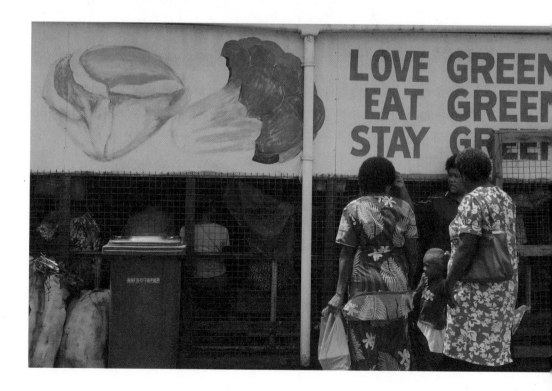

bean sprouts are a rich source of amino acids, fiber, vitamins and minerals, and also helpful in enhancing iron absorption of the other ingredients in the meal. Stir-fry or eat raw in salads. Bean sprouts stay fresh for about two days, so freeze them when you come back from the market and defrost in a pan of cold water when needed — you could even grow your own.

bell peppers are a powerful force in the produce aisle: beautiful to look at, full of disease-fighting antioxidants and delicious to taste both cooked and raw. Also known as a "capsicum," a green pepper turns red when left longer on the vine to ripen (becoming sweeter). Many herbalists recommend this native American vegetable as a natural metabolism enhancer due to its role in lowering triglycerides. Choose blemish-free peppers and refrigerate in an airtight container for up to 5 days. Preserve by dipping in boiling water for 30 seconds, slice thinly and freeze.

berries are a natural weight-loss remedy, with insoluble fiber content similar to bran and whole grain cereals! You'll save loads of money if you buy them while they are in season and freeze (they only last a couple of days in the fridge). Place flat on a baking tray for a few hours in the freezer, then store in an airtight container. Frozen berries make tasty after-dinner treats!

black beans have similar antioxidants amounts to grapes and cranberries, are packed with fiber and are a high-quality protein source when combined with whole grains such as brown rice. Dry and canned are available year-round in the bulk food aisle at your local supermarket. We only use a small amount on this diet, so most find it more practical to use an organic canned variety.

broccoli is rich in calcium and vitamin C. When you come home from the market, cover the broccoli that you need for the next couple of days in plastic wrap and store in the fridge. Cook the rest of the broccoli in boiling water for a minute or so, cut into small florets and freeze in an airtight container.

carrots Just one small carrot per day has enough vitamin A to improve your vision and protect against cancer! You can meet this quota by snacking on baby carrots, grating carrot into your rice or drinking in a juice blend. Cooked carrots contain higher nutritional benefits than raw as the beta-carotene is absorbed more easily. Cut off the leafy tops before storing for maximum vitamin retention.

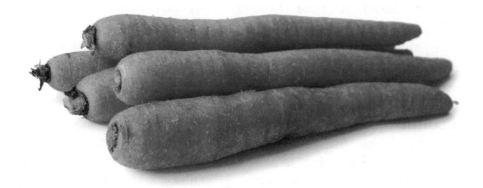

chickpeas (garbanzo beans) are excellent for the heart and assist in preventing cardiovascular disease. They are very high in fiber and protein, stabilizing blood sugar levels by slowing digestion and increasing nutrient absorption. They are nutty in texture and are popular in Middle Eastern and Indian recipes. As the recipes only require a small amount, use the organic canned variety and freeze what you don't use.

celery is a great post-workout crunch as it is high in minerals and helps replace lost electrolytes with naturally occurring sodium (the good kind). It can help relieve constipation due to its laxative effect, cut salt cravings and curb appetite between meals — making it a great snack for weight loss. Keep celery crisp by refrigerating in airtight container. Enjoy cooked or raw.

cilantro (coriander) helps weight loss as it has been known to reduce the body's absorption of saturated fat. Daily use promotes clear, radiant skin and reduced risk of skin cancer due to its ability to trap the free radicals caused by exposure to the sun. Fresh cilantro lasts a week: when you come home from the market, choose the best leaves, wash and cut ends off the stem. Arrange in cool water (change the water every few days) and keep in the fridge.

coconut flakes are used in the fish-coating recipes. New studies show that coconut fats (medium-chain triglycerides) produce energy much faster than other saturated fats, which actually raises your metabolism. Researchers say this is partly due to it being absorbed by the liver instead of being stored in fat cells.

corn has been cultivated by farmers for over 10,000 years. This cereal grain is a sweet-tasting complex carbohydrate, high in minerals such as potassium, zinc and iron — great for vegans as it has high vitamin B12 and folic acid content. Corn is high in calories, making it a valuable energy supply in developing nations.

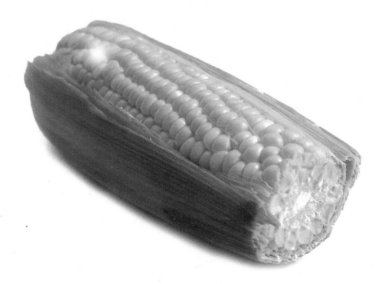

cucumber is low in calories, known to promote radiant skin due to its silica content. Place on your eyes as a beauty treatment! Naturally hydrating, cucumber helps to reduce blood pressure and water retention. Choose cucumbers displayed in refrigerators as they are sensitive to heat. Buy organic when possible as supermarket varieties are often waxed.

edamame (ed-ah-mah-mey) is the Japanese word used to describe boiled green soybean. They can be used to replace lima beans in any dish. You'll love this sweet, crunchy treat — it's got loads of antioxidants, nutrients, fiber and more protein than 4 slices of bacon. Find them in the frozen foods section, shelled or still in the pod. Shelled edamame is a popular snack as you have to pop each one and eat consciously. Unshelled are most convenient for cooking. Look for non-GMO soybeans to ensure they are organic.

garlic Buy garlic once a week to keep it fresh — use the fattest cloves of the bulb and store at room temperature with its top attached so it stays pungent. Garlic is a natural antibiotic that also helps lower blood sugar levels, making it a great choice for diabetics.

ginger is a light spice, high in natural enzymes that can help you absorb the nutrients of your meal. It can be used with any combination of spices to add a mellow sweetness, as both a sauté and garnish. Adding ginger to the black bean recipe makes the beans more digestible, preventing gas. It's also a natural mood enhancer — drink ginger tea anytime.

green beans have similar nutritional benefits to lima, black or kidney beans, except they can be eaten both raw or cooked. They're low in calories and high in iron — a great snack choice. Choose bright beans that are skinnier than a pencil.

jalapeño pepper Learn to love it! *The Planet Friendly Diet* uses lots of jalapeño because of its thermogenic properties that increase your fat-burning ability and metabolism. It's hot and spicy, so build your tolerance up gradually! The red peppers that you'll use in the salsa tend to be sweet — choose brightly colored peppers and store unwrapped in the fridge.

lemons make everything taste clean! They are one of the most import-ant fruits to have in the kitchen — use freely as a sour, acidic zest to any recipe or drink. Lemons are so powerful from a nutritional standpoint that if you have health conditions like heartburn, gall bladder stones, kidney stones or citrus allergy, you will need to ask your doctor prior to using lemon juice.

Lemon juice is fully packed with nutrients like vitamin C, vitamin B complex, fiber, calcium, iron and magnesium. It's acidic in nature, but once it gets into the body and mixes with stomach's secretions, its effect become alkaline. It can have some detrimental effects on tooth enamel. Lemon juice should be diluted with lukewarm water instead of very hot or cold water to get maximum results.

Lemon has been acclaimed for its health benefits for centuries. It helps to reduce stress, boost immunity, increase weight loss, detoxify the body, kill harmful microorganisms and increase bowel movements which in turn helps fight against intestinal diseases like constipation. Its detoxification and weight-loss properties are based on the high levels of glutathione pres-ent, an antioxidant. Studies on mouse white adipose tissues have revealed that lemon can supress the fat accumulation in the body and weight gain. It also contains pectin fiber that will help in fighting against hunger cravings, and therefore it will stop you from overeating. Lemon peel also has a good effect on heart health as its use can decrease cholesterol in plasma and in

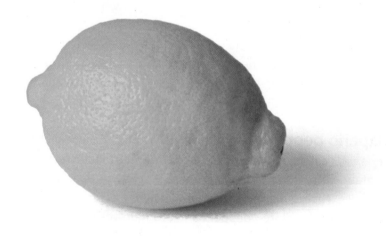

the liver; also that is why it can reduce the risk of many heart diseases. It also contains K+ ions that are necessary for rhythmic heart contractions. Need more Vitamin C? Lemons are loaded with it. Vitamin C is the main constituent of platelets, which helps in blood clotting; lemon juice can increase platelet count, which will help you in fast clotting of blood should you get into an accident and have excessive bleeding. Lemon juice can also help to fight against various diseases like dengue fever and scurvy.

Lemons have an atomic structure similar to saliva and hydrochloric acid secreted by the stomach; they stimulate the production of bile and other enzymes from the liver. Not only does it boost digestion, lemon juice is also a diuretic that helps flush out toxins and alleviate headaches. Squeeze several throughout the day into lukewarm water to detox and flush your colon, increase energy, reduce swelling and balance your body's pH levels. Store lemons at room temperature.

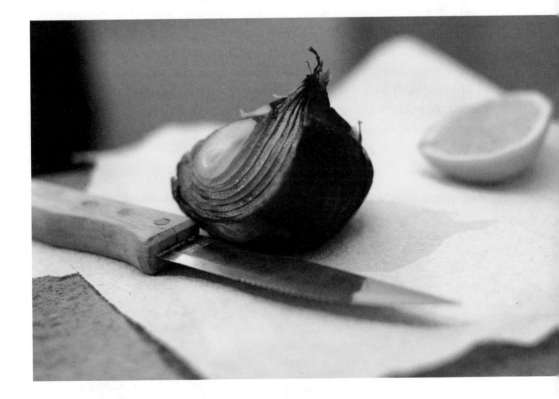

lettuce is a great way to freshen up a dish. Store for up to a week in a plastic bag in the fridge after removing the core (smash down on the kitchen counter) and rinsing the head under cold water.

mango is delicious cooked or raw. It is a true super-food with powerful antioxidant properties that can help clear up your skin, boost digestion and protect against heart disease. This iron-rich tropical fruit can be enjoyed anytime as a snack or blended into smoothies.

mushrooms are great if you are craving meat or fries! Sauté them in a pan with a handful of spinach and a sprinkle of sesame seeds for an anytime snack. If you buy your mushrooms at a farmers' market, buy from a well-known vendor. Mushrooms can be highly poisonous! So avoid discolored mushrooms — pick individually at the supermarket (pre-sliced is an unnecessary way to increase your grocery cost). Refrigerate unprepped in a brown paper bag.

onions vary in color, flavor and use, but all are a low-calorie way to spice up a meal. Use onions in small amounts while on this diet as they are an appetite stimulant — many restaurants load your plate in hopes that you'll eat more. Store at room temperature in a cool, dry place — they will keep for weeks.

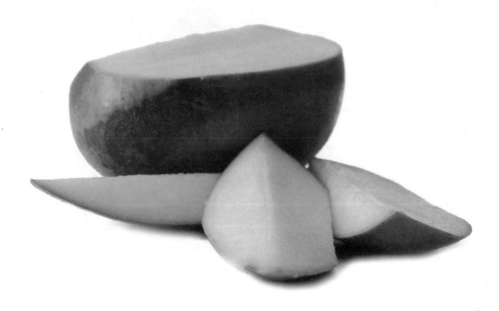

orange juice (and juices in general) can be unnecessary sources of sugar and calories... however, adding a little to your smoothie gives it a welcome zing, especially if you juice it yourself. Juicing is the healthiest and freshest option compared to store-bought; however, if you're buying OJ from the store, pick a juice with lots of pulp as that's where the fiber is. Anything that says fruit "drink" in the name is not real juice and will be full of sugar. Juices with a shorter shelf life are the most natural and free of preservatives. At *Whistler Fitness Vacations*, we make orange cubes by pouring the juice into an ice cube tray to help portion control (4 cubes is half a cup).

potatoes have long been thought of as a fattening starch — this is false! Potatoes are a heart-healthy food, high in fiber and potassium. For best potassium retention, bake for about 45 minutes or steam them. Pick potatoes individually so you can check for discolorations and firmness (better than bulk buying in a sack). Store potatoes in a paper or cloth bag at room temperature, away from apples.

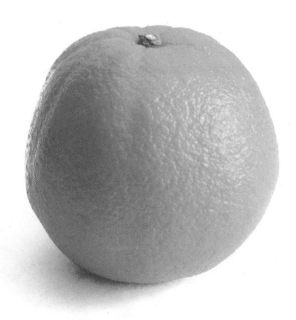

protein powder When choosing a protein powder, avoid artificial colors or flavors, preservatives, pesticides, sweeteners, eggs and gluten. Vegan powder (found at most health food stores and some pharmacies) is usually the best choice as it is easiest to digest, blends well with other ingredients and has the most minimal taste. This is good because you taste the fresh fruit that you add to it — not the powder.

quinoa contains more protein than any other grain. It's a good source of dietary fiber, phosphorous, calcium, vitamin E, magnesium, potassium and iron. Quinoa is gluten-free and easy to digest due to its almost perfect balance of all 8 essential amino acids— which are needed for tissue development in humans.

red cabbage has a hearty strong flavor and is more nutritionally dense than green cabbage — with almost 8 times more vitamin C per serving. Choose cabbage heads that are shiny, crisp and firm: ask your grocer to cut it in half if only whole cabbages are displayed. Red cabbage keeps in your fridge for a week or so — cover tightly with plastic wrap.

sesame seeds can be found in the bulk food or cooking aisle. Historians believe they may be the world's oldest condiment (dating back to 1600 BC). These little seeds pack a punch: sprinkle a teaspoon on any meal for added iron, dietary fiber and calcium (for about 25 calories).

snap peas are bright, crispy and sweet with lots of lots of vitamin A, C and K. Look for the rounded pod (the snow pea is flatter). Wash well, chop off the ends and eat the whole pea, including the outer skin. These are popular raw or cooked — toss in a stir-fry or have plain as a crunchy snack. Snap peas keep for a week or more when refrigerated.

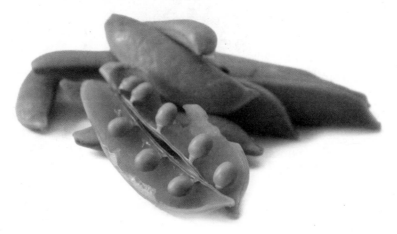

soy milk is complete protein containing no cholesterol or saturated fat. This makes it good for your bones, muscles and arteries. If you are intolerant to soy or just prefer not to use it, use rice, almond or coconut milk as an alternative. Just a heads-up however: almond and rice milk have quite a sweet texture that doesn't make them as versatile for cooking. Rice milk is also lower in protein.

There are several controversies surrounding the safety of soy and whether it should be used as part of a *Planet Friendly Diet*. The FDA monitors all food products and states that the hormones in soy-based food products are safe, but many argue that is not the case. One concern (and the reason that many link it to increased risk of breast cancer) is due to the estrogen association of the isoflavones present, which can bind to certain receptors that may act like estrogen on the body. Although this may be valid to a point, isoflavones also provide many positive effects on the body, including cellular growth that in fact protects against many cancers, in addition to keeping cholesterol levels in check due to its fiber content. Asia has one of the lowest rates of breast cancer in the world and has one of the highest consumption of soy-based products. Risks of animal-based estrogen are much higher than using soybean products. Another concern is the effect on heart health and thyroid. Scientists have found that isoflavones taken daily have been useful in lowering blood pressure, making it in fact good for your heart. Concerns about thyroid are only valid for those with an existing thyroid problem (especially those taking medications for it) because soy products can interfere with the effectiveness of the medication. Speak with your doctor for guidance — you can still enjoy soy products while on thyroid medication but just take them a few hours apart.

The bottom line about soy is to consume it in moderation.

Use whole or fermented soy foods only. It's not dangerous or unhealthy if you treat it like a treat, a couple of times a week but perhaps not everyday. Read the labels and select the purest forms of soy products — not processed, as the nutrients are stripped. If it says "soy protein" on the label, don't buy it. Choose soy milk that is fresh, has an upcoming expiry date and is made from whole beans with no added flavoring or sugars. Don't be afraid of edamame (young soybeans) — while the dishes in *The Planet Friendly Diet* use lima beans, you can safely and happily switch them out for organic soybeans. In fact, the photos are taken with soybeans; they're a great source of protein and have awesome levels of probiotics. Miso is also a safe, healthy choice as it's rich in vitamin B12 and a really good metabolic booster. Just choose the low-sodium variety.

spinach contains more iron per gram than a ground hamburger patty. Adding vitamin C and calcium to your spinach dish can increase iron absorption. This green leafy veggie can be best purchased frozen if it is out of season, as the nutritional benefits get quickly lost after it is picked. Even if you keep spinach in the fridge, it will lose valuable vitamins and minerals after just 4 days. So take a look at what you need right away and preserve the rest in the freezer. Dip spinach in boiling water for 30 seconds, cover each individual portion with plastic wrap and freeze.

tofu Spiced-up tofu is delicious and nutritious — it absorbs the flavor of surrounding ingredients and plays the main role in many meat-free meals. This traditional Asian food was developed over 2,000 years ago by the Chinese and is smooth in texture. Choose the extra-firm variety — take what you need for the week and freeze the rest. If you have intolerance to soy products, you can substitute egg whites, chickpeas, kidney beans or white fish.

tomatoes have long been favored as a cancer-fighting antioxidant due to their powerful healing properties. Big round ones add unbeatable freshness to almost any meal, with their cherry cousin a sweet variation. Stock up on tomatoes while they are in season — when you get home from the market, dip them into boiling water for about 30 seconds, chop and freeze in recipe-size portions.

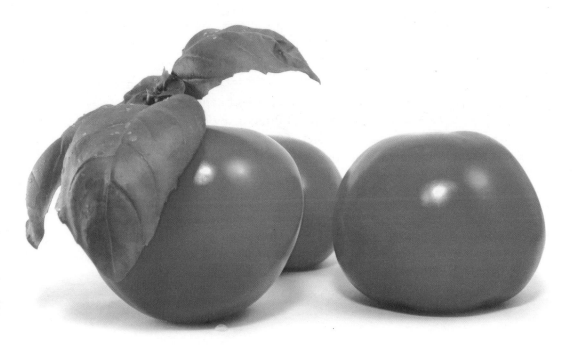

yogurt can be dairy-free! While soy yogurt is the most common dairy-free option, there are several alternatives available. Ricera makes a rice milk yogurt that is casein, soy, wheat and gluten-free, and So Delicious makes one with cultured coconut milk. All dairy-free yogurts are nutritious, high in calcium and good for the digestive system. Try a few kinds or make your own. Buy larger containers to save money and packaging (check expiry date).

zucchini is a summer squash, also known as a courgette. It grows year-round and can be eaten raw, cooked or grilled. The smaller younger zucchini are the sweetest and most flavorful — the slender firm ones are the best. Zucchinis are high in water content (95%), which is helpful in restricting calories as it makes you feel full. For later use, cook in boiling water for a couple of minutes, cool and freeze in an airtight bag.

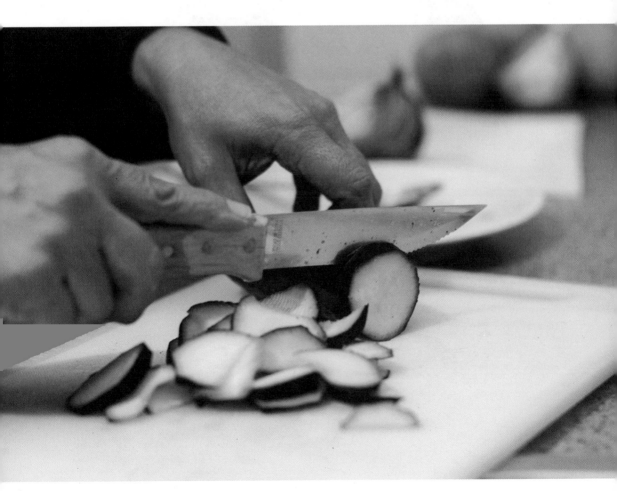

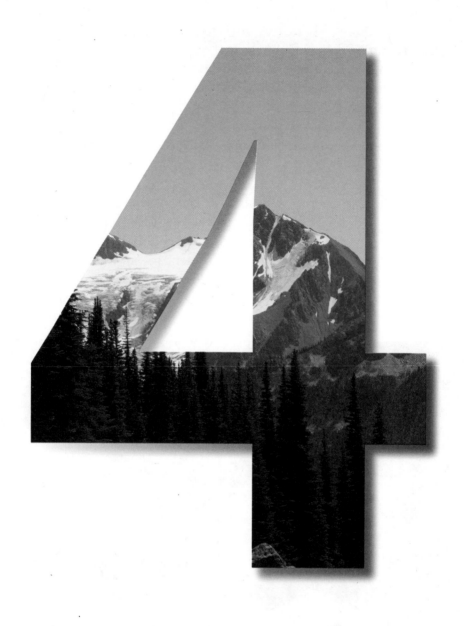

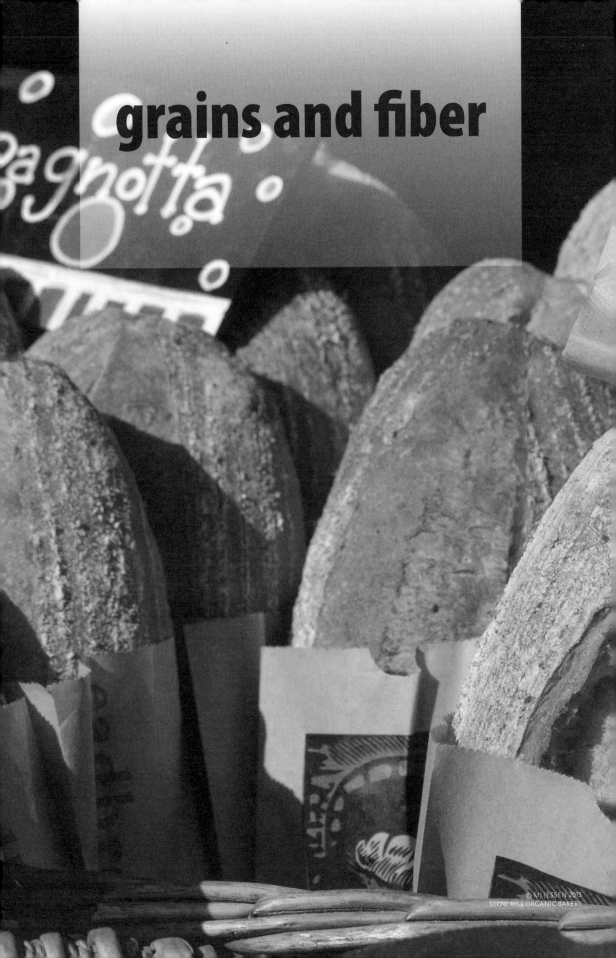

grains and fiber

© M.J ESSEN 2015
SLOW RISE ORGANIC BAKERY

whole grains

Whole grains or foods made from them still have all the essential parts and naturally occurring nutrients of the entire grain seed. All parts of the grain kernel (cereal germ, endosperm and bran) must be present to qualify as whole grain. This grain may be cracked, crushed, rolled, extruded or cooked through processing and will still deliver the full benefits of the whole grain fiber, iron, calcium and B vitamins. Whole grains also help with the immune system in addition to the development of healthy bones, as they provide a great source of magnesium and selenium. Identify whole grain products by the ingredient list — if the nutritional information lists whole wheat, whole meal or whole corn as the first ingredient, the product is a whole grain food item. If the product says enriched, wheat flour or whole wheat flour, the product is likely not a whole grain content. The fiber in whole wheat and whole grain products allow the food's energy to enter your bloodstream at a slower rate, which translates into sustainable long-term energy, keeping you fuller for longer.

tip nº 30

eat whole grains

Whole grains are cereal grains such as amaranth, barley, buckwheat, corn, millet, oats and oatmeal, brown rice, rye, wheat — including spelt, emmer, farro, einkorn, kamut, durum and forms such as bulgar, cracked wheat and wheatberries. These ingredients make healthy products, including whole grain breads, pastas, rolled oats (porridge) and oat groats, and are a natural source of protein and complex carbohydrate. "Multigrain" is another confusing term that includes a multitude of grain products that do not necessarily contain the endosperm, cereal germ and bran that you need.

Whole meal products are made from whole grain flour. Some food manufacturers make foods with whole grain ingredients ("contains whole grain"); however, unless it is listed as the first ingredient, it should not be considered a whole grain food product.

tip nº 31

wheat makes you hungry

whole wheat grains are the good guys. They contain the whole grain of wheat.

wheat grains have the bran and germ removed during the "refining process." Almost half of the nutrients of wheat flour are stripped away, drastically reducing the B vitamins and fiber intake, which in turn will drastically reduce your bowel movement. When constipated for a while, you may feel sluggish and toxic — perhaps even get a headache or start to feel depressed. This may be because the undigested portions of wheat are fermenting inside, leaking to the bloodstream and spiking insulin levels. Spiked blood sugar levels usually lead to increased hunger.

Some experts estimate that up to 70% of the population suffer from intolerance to wheat without realizing it. Unfortunately, digestive disorders often go undiagnosed. Whole grain is a better choice for diabetics especially.

 action step

Eat foods from this list, as they indicate healthy whole grain products:

- whole wheat bread
- whole wheat buns/rolls

- whole wheat macaroni, spaghetti or vermicelli
- cracked wheat
- crushed wheat
- entire wheat flour
- bromated wheat
- whole durum flour
- bulgar wheat

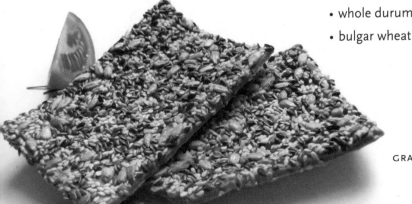

tip nº 32

add vitamin C to pulses and grains

Pulses lack the amino acid that grains have and vice versa. When you combine the two, you create a complete protein, but you need to take it one step further if you are going to maintain healthy iron levels.

As most meat eaters will tell you, vegetarians run the risk of dipping low in energy and iron if they don't understand the science of plant-protein combining. The formula is really very simple — add vitamin C to your grains and pulses so that you'll absorb enough iron from your vegetarian meal to protect from iron-deficiency anemia and maintain healthy metabolism. It is the B vitamins thiamin, riboflavin and niacin that help burn calories from your protein, fat and carbohydrates (also help your nervous system), so adding fresh tomatoes, green leafy vegetables or fruit to your grains and pulses is really important for many reasons.

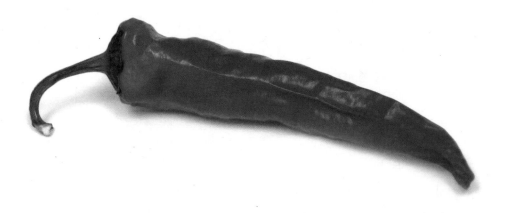

tip no 33

learn to read food labels

Choose foods that name one of the following whole grain ingredients first on the label's ingredient list: brown rice, buckwheat, bulgur, millet, oatmeal, quinoa, rolled oats, whole grain barley, whole grain corn, whole grain sorghum, whole grain triticale, whole oats, whole rye, whole wheat, wild rice. Foods labeled with the words multigrain, stone-ground, 100% wheat, cracked wheat, seven-grain or bran are usually not whole grain products.

Color is not an indication of a whole grain. Bread can be brown because of molasses or other added ingredients. Read the ingredient list to see if it is a whole grain. Use the Nutrition Facts label and choose whole grain products with a higher percentage daily value (% DV) for fiber. Most whole grain products are great sources of fiber.

Read the food label's ingredient list. Look for terms that indicate added sugars (such as sucrose, high-fructose corn syrup, honey, malt syrup, maple syrup, molasses or raw sugar) that add extra calories. Choose foods with fewer added sugars.

Most sodium in the food supply comes from packaged foods. Similar packaged foods can vary widely in sodium content, including breads. Use the Nutrition Facts label to choose foods with a lower % DV for sodium. Look for foods labeled "low in sodium," as that indicates they have less than 140 mg sodium per serving.

tip № 34

stay away from refined grains

Refined grains are "food-like products" with the same amount of calories as nutritious foods, but with all the nutrition stripped.

They are often disguised as health food, which easily misleads the consumer into believing that what they are eating is a valuable part of their diet. Refined grain products are white pasta, white rice and white bread.

action steps

- When baking, substitute half of the all-purpose white flour with whole wheat flour. You'll barely notice the difference.

- Air-popped popcorn is a great whole grain choice. Filling and low in fat! For a bit more flavor, sprinkle with a tablespoon of grated parmesan cheese or a dash of sea salt.

- When cooking stir-fry, set the prepared stir-fry on a beautiful bed of brown rice. It takes a little longer to cook than white rice, so plan to cook the brown rice while you prepare other elements of the meal.

- If making cookies, add some oatmeal. A great whole grain!

- When making pasta dishes, use whole grain pasta. It's delicious and takes the same amount of time to cook.

- Try different grains such as quinoa or bulgur. They are a breeze to make and taste delicious and a little nutty.

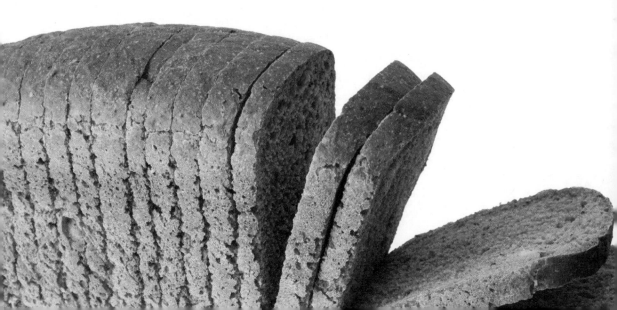

tip nº 35

poop twice a day

The Planet Friendly Diet is a cleansing detox diet designed to give you 2 or 3 bowel movements per day. If you are not having this, move to oatmeal in the morning instead of the smoothie and check fiber intake to bring it to 25 grams per day. Bowel movement is when stools are expelled from the body after food is absorbed in the gastrointestinal tract; the remaining undigested food and waste products are present in our stool.

To maintain optimal health, our body needs to defecate unnecessary substances, which is why there must be certain number of bowel movements in a day. More than 3 is a condition known as diarrhoea, in which stools mainly consist of water; and less than 2 is constipation, which makes you feel pain and difficulty in passing hard stools, as there is less water present.

If you don't eat whole grain, you'll likely become constipated as minimal fiber requirements won't be met. Additional contributing factors to constipation include not getting enough water and exercise. Constipated people miss the opportunity to remove about 200 calories of waste every day in the bathroom (based on 9 calories being removed from your body per gram of insoluble fiber eaten). This is one of the reasons why it's so important to get your bowel movements on track if you're trying to lose weight. Even if you're gluten, wheat and barley intolerant, there are plenty of products out there to give your body the endosperm, cereal germ and bran combination that it needs to clean out and detoxify.

There are health-related issues associated with chronic (prolonged) diarrhoea that may include different cancers, haemorrhoids, arthritis, obesity and diverticulitis; or it can be a symptom of diseases like multiple sclerosis, Parkinson's disease, hypothyroidism, depression, colorectal cancer and irritable bowel syndrome. People who don't have healthy bowel movements feel toxic, malnourished, sick and exhausted. Switching up your diet by following recommendations in *The Planet Friendly Diet* is more holistic and healthier than laxatives and fiber pills.

reduce gluten

Gluten is the protein in wheat that allows dough to rise and bind, but while the glue-like substance makes beautiful bread, it is often rejected by our digestive system. This can cause bacteria growth, reducing the absorption rate of calcium, vitamin A and iron.

Gluten-free is the buzz word these days, used to process grains that naturally have gluten in them, like wheat (spelt, kamut, durum, farro, bulgur, barley, rye and semolina), and the food industry is trying hard to rebuild, rebrand and reboot their products as a healthy alternative to the regular brands offering full gluten ingredients. There are whole grain products that naturally don't have gluten in them — these are a better choice than products that have been processed to be able to show a "gluten-free" label.

Your best bet is to stick to foods that don't naturally have gluten in them, like brown rice. More than 40,000 different varieties are cultivated in over 100 countries on every continent except Antartica, so it's very likely you'll be able to source it reasonably locally. In fact, 96% of the rice eaten is eaten in the area where it is grown. Thailand, Vietnam, India and the USA are the top 4 rice-exporting countries in the world. Other naturally gluten-free grains include amaranth, buckwheat, corn, millet, quinoa and oats that haven't been around wheat during growing or processing.

Wheat has been grown for over 10 thousand years, but massive demand has meant that the farming and cultivation methods have become greatly compromised. With increased pesticides and so forth, intolerance is on the rise. If you've gone through *The Planet Friendly Diet* for 21 days without adding oatmeal for breakfast or having gluten-based snacks and you have no side effects eating a whole grain sandwich on Day 22, then you're probably not gluten intolerant. What gives gluten a bad rap is primarily that the excessive consumption of overeating plays havoc with your intestinal system, with discomforts such as joint inflammation, bloating, irritability, skin rashes, diarrhea, constipation, acid reflux, unexplained iron deficiency. Stick with real foods that are naturally gluten-free, as much as you can.

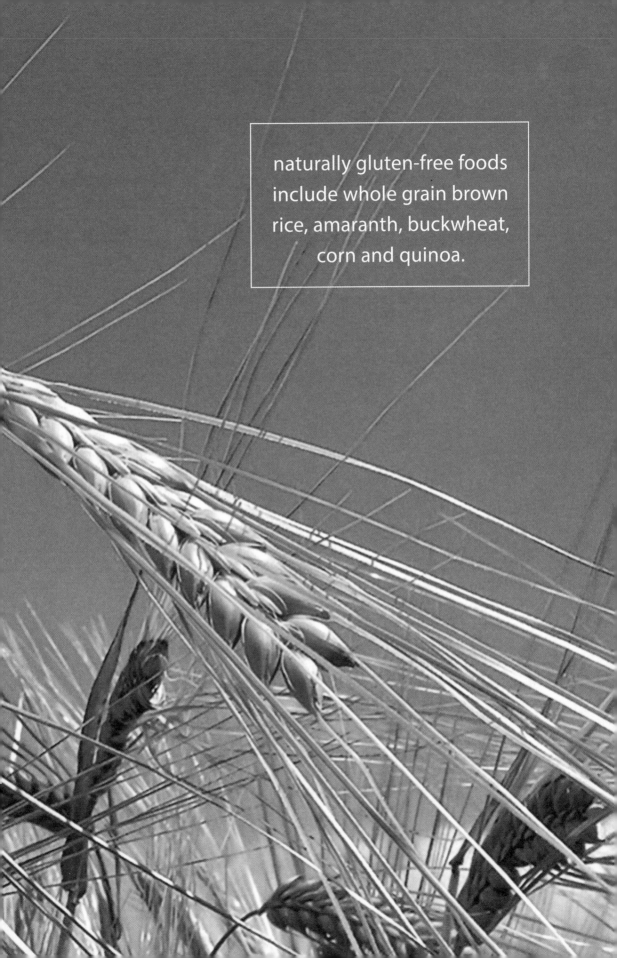

naturally gluten-free foods include whole grain brown rice, amaranth, buckwheat, corn and quinoa.

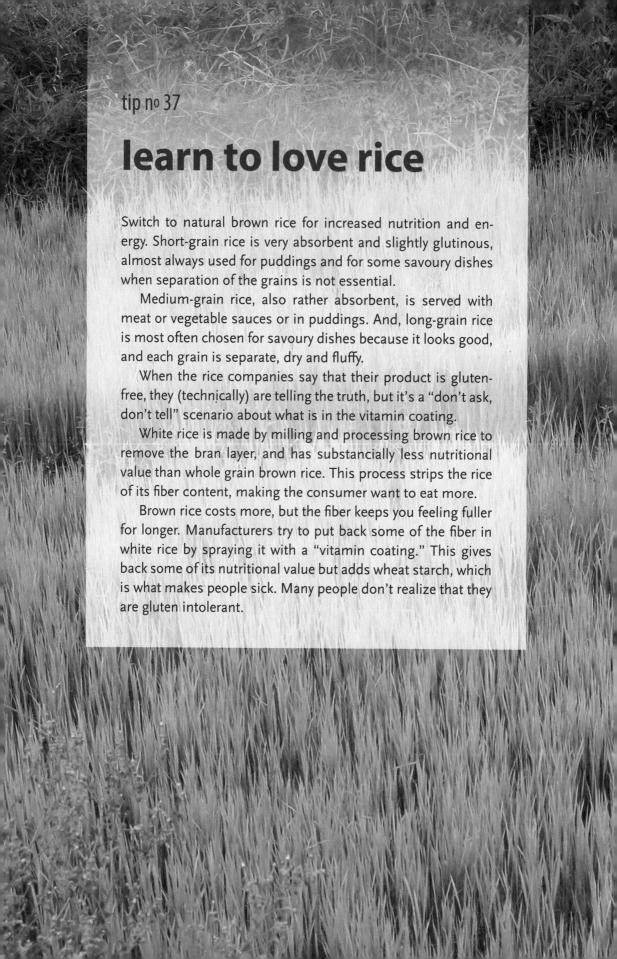

tip n⁰ 37

learn to love rice

Switch to natural brown rice for increased nutrition and energy. Short-grain rice is very absorbent and slightly glutinous, almost always used for puddings and for some savoury dishes when separation of the grains is not essential.

Medium-grain rice, also rather absorbent, is served with meat or vegetable sauces or in puddings. And, long-grain rice is most often chosen for savoury dishes because it looks good, and each grain is separate, dry and fluffy.

When the rice companies say that their product is gluten-free, they (technically) are telling the truth, but it's a "don't ask, don't tell" scenario about what is in the vitamin coating.

White rice is made by milling and processing brown rice to remove the bran layer, and has substancially less nutritional value than whole grain brown rice. This process strips the rice of its fiber content, making the consumer want to eat more.

Brown rice costs more, but the fiber keeps you feeling fuller for longer. Manufacturers try to put back some of the fiber in white rice by spraying it with a "vitamin coating." This gives back some of its nutritional value but adds wheat starch, which is what makes people sick. Many people don't realize that they are gluten intolerant.

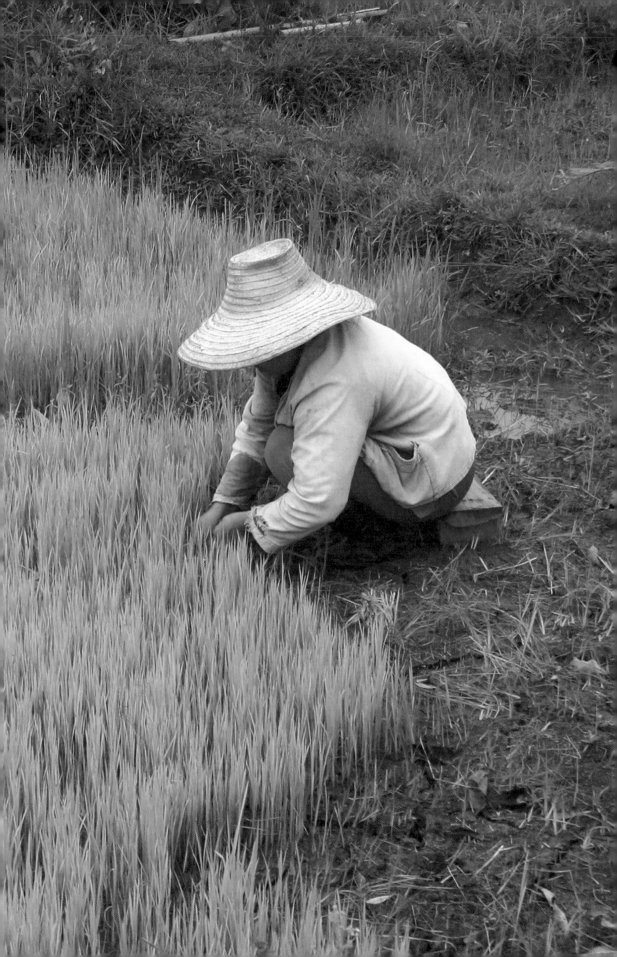

tip no 38

toppings add up

We often overcompensate for the blandness of the grain products by slathering on fatty spreads and sauces. You can still eat your favourite foods, but you need to make a compromise. Try low-fat cream, or instead of butter, try a light smear of peanut butter.

Choose low-sugar, low-fat, whole grain cereals. If you feel these choices are bland, a sprinkling of sugar is fine, as long as it is limited to a teaspoon. "Whole grain" Fruit Loops, Lucky Charms and such are not what they assume to be — it is not whole grain unless the first ingredient is whole grain, and even then they are packed with sugar, food coloring, additives and preservatives.

portion sizes

We only need between 7 and 10 servings of whole grain products per day. This may seem like a lot; one portion may be less than you think! Examples of one serving of grain products:

- 1 slice of bread
- ½ of a 12-inch pita bread or tortilla
- ½ cup of cooked rice, quinoa or bulgur
- 30 g of cereal (measurement in cups of cereals depends on the puffiness of the cereal. Look at the nutritional information on the box to get an idea of how many cups equal a serving.)
- ¾ cup of hot cereal such as oatmeal
- ½ cup whole grain pasta

Restaurants often serve up to 5 portions in one serving — half a cup of pasta fits into the palm of your hand.

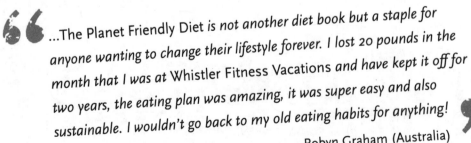

...The Planet Friendly Diet is not another diet book but a staple for anyone wanting to change their lifestyle forever. I lost 20 pounds in the month that I was at Whistler Fitness Vacations and have kept it off for two years, the eating plan was amazing, it was super easy and also sustainable. I wouldn't go back to my old eating habits for anything!
— Robyn Graham (Australia)

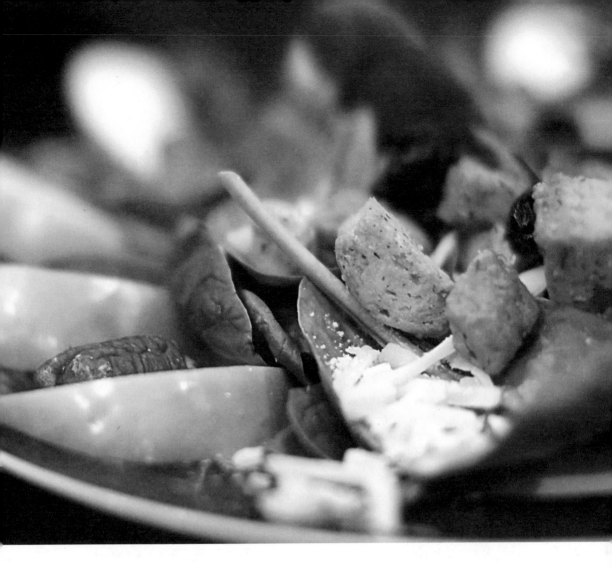

action steps

Some tips for keeping the amounts of grain product consumption within a reasonable range:

- At mealtime, eat open-faced sandwiches and burgers.

- When dining out at the restaurant, avoid the bread basket. It's okay to feel a little hungry while waiting for your main course to arrive. Ask the waiter to remove the bread basket from the table.

- Don't coat bread in butter or sugary jams, or immerse in oil.

- Make pasta a side dish of your meal. Serve pasta with a protein and some vegetables. You can enjoy pasta in smaller amounts.

- When eating at a restaurant, request a half-portion of pasta or share it with a friend. Even that is much more than the recommended serving for two.

- Prepare pastas with non-creamy sauces such as tomato sauce or a little bit of basil pesto.

nature doesn't need to be enriched (or fortified)

When you learn how to eat a balanced diet, you will get all the vitamins and minerals that you need. Keep foods in their natural state so that your digestive system doesn't overload with foreign substances. Do you want an orange or sugar-free pop with vitamin C added? Go natural!

enriched means that nutrients were lost during processing, therefore they were added by artificial means afterwards. For example, enriched wheat flour means that the white flour had fiber products and vitamins added to it to give nutritional characteristic similar to the whole wheat.

fortified signifies that nutrients that the food did not naturally have were added during processing. For example, calcium, vitamin D and vitamin B12 fortified soy products. As soy products don't naturally contain much calcium, adding calcium makes people who are used to drinking milk more comfortable with switching to soy milk. This is not necessary, however, as calcium can be found in the same place as cows find it — green leafy produce from the ground.

action step

The daily recommended Intake for fiber is 25 g, with an upper limit of 40 g. If you are starting to increase your fiber intake, do it slowly.

A drastic increase will make you bloated and uncomfortable. Drink lots of water to keep things transporting smoothly.

complex carbs include starches and fibers. Whole grain bread products, brown rice, whole grain pasta, cereals and potatoes are sources of complex carbs in our diets. As fiber goes through the digestive system, it soaks up liquid like a sponge, increasing in bulk, with the digestive juices penetrating the fiber that consequently extracts the nutrients. This takes time, which is why complex carbs take longer to absorb into the system than simple carbs.

soluble fiber is the supportive structure of all cereals, fruit and vegetables. It's been associated with protection against heart disease and diabetes, due to its ability to bind to cholesterol and lower blood glucose levels. Soluble fiber is commonly found in legumes (beans and peas) and fruits. Plain oatmeal is a great source of soluble fiber. Soluble fiber is also excellent for weight loss and weight control, as it forms a gel when being digested. This makes you feel fuller longer, preventing you from overeating.

insoluble fiber is most recognizable as bran and does not form a gel in your gastrointestinal tract. It is not digested by your body, and therefore acts as an "intestinal broom" — meaning it'll help clear you out. In fact, every gram of insoluble fiber consumed removes 9 calories from your daily calorie total. This does not mean that a fiber-containing food is calorie free; it is, however, low in calories and an awesome choice.

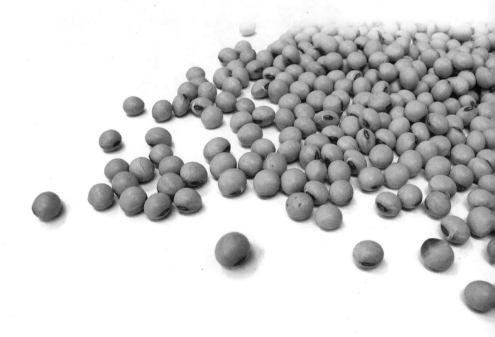

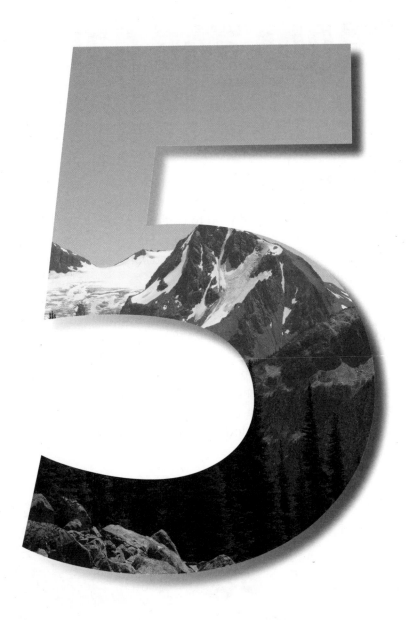

eggs and dairy

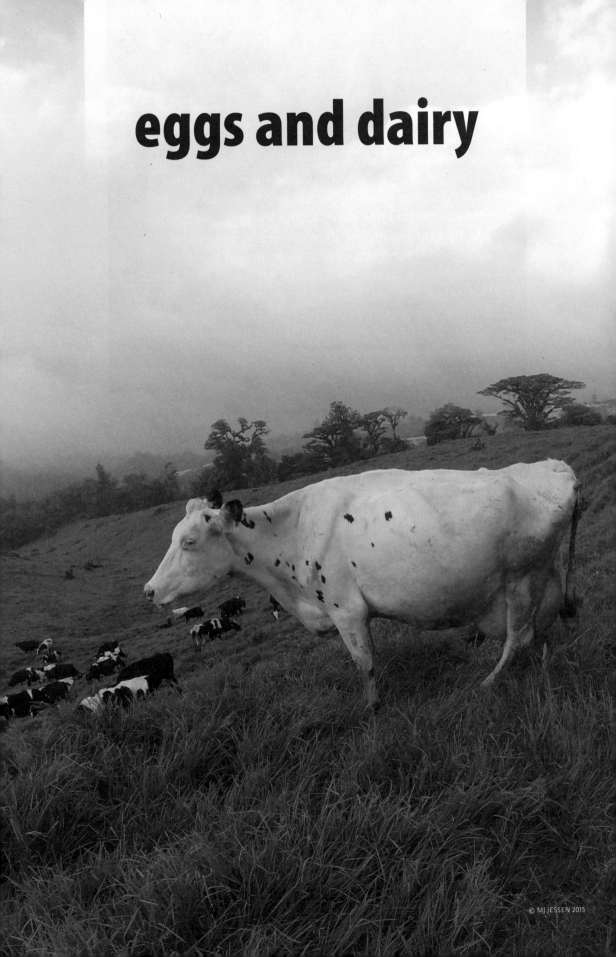

eggs

Eggs are power-packed with protein, fat and iron plus vitamins A, D, E, B2 and B12. These vitamins are great for your eyesight, producing red blood cells, protecting from disease and breaking down food into energy. Vitamins A and B2 help growth and development in children. Whole eggs can help you lose weight — according to a study by the Rochester Center for Obesity Research. They found that those who ate eggs for breakfast ate 400 calories less the rest of the day compared to people who did not eat eggs. Eggs can keep you fuller for longer due to the balance they provide, the essential amino acids, iron, zinc and phosphorus.

action step

The smart way to eat eggs and save calories is to eat one whole egg (80 calories) and toss the yolks of the other eggs used — just be sure to eat calcium and iron-rich foods during the day. For example, scramble 4 egg whites (15 calories each) with sautéed mushrooms and spinach and serve with fresh salsa on some whole wheat toast for a delicious 300-calorie breakfast. It's all about the planning and budgeting of calories — only eating what you can afford.

tip no 40

give the yolks to your dog

One medium egg has about 80 calories and 6 grams of protein, which can quickly add up. Two eggs "cost" 160 calories, so by the time you add toast, butter and a bit of cheese, you're looking at a 500-calorie breakfast... and that's not counting your latte. Yolk has over 90% of an egg's calcium and iron, and the white has almost half the egg's protein.

tip nº 41

choose organic free-range eggs

Eating planet friendly means reducing consumption of animal products and by-products. Almost all of North America's egg-laying hens live in tiny wire cubes packed with up to 7 birds, stacked up in rows in barns without windows. Their beaks are cut to stop them from fighting, and their entire life is about laying eggs.

Choose organic free-range eggs from hens that have been raised humanely. Farmers are only able to get their organic stamp if they pass animal welfare standards — right down to using food without antibiotics and growth hormones. Don't be fooled by "fed vegetarian feed" or "omega rich." Spend a few extra dimes and buy eggs that do not support battery hen operations.

Cage-free eggs means that the hens are not packed into a battery cage. The hens remain inside throughout their lives, and you have no assurance over what kind of medication they are given to produce eggs.

Free-run eggs means the birds move around in bigger barns; however, they may not have access to outside, and there are usually many birds jammed into the barn.

Free-range eggs means that the hens have been allowed to go outside and put their feet on the ground.

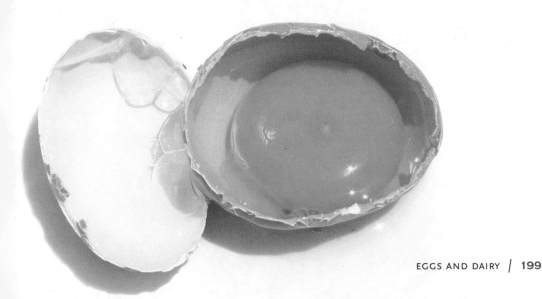

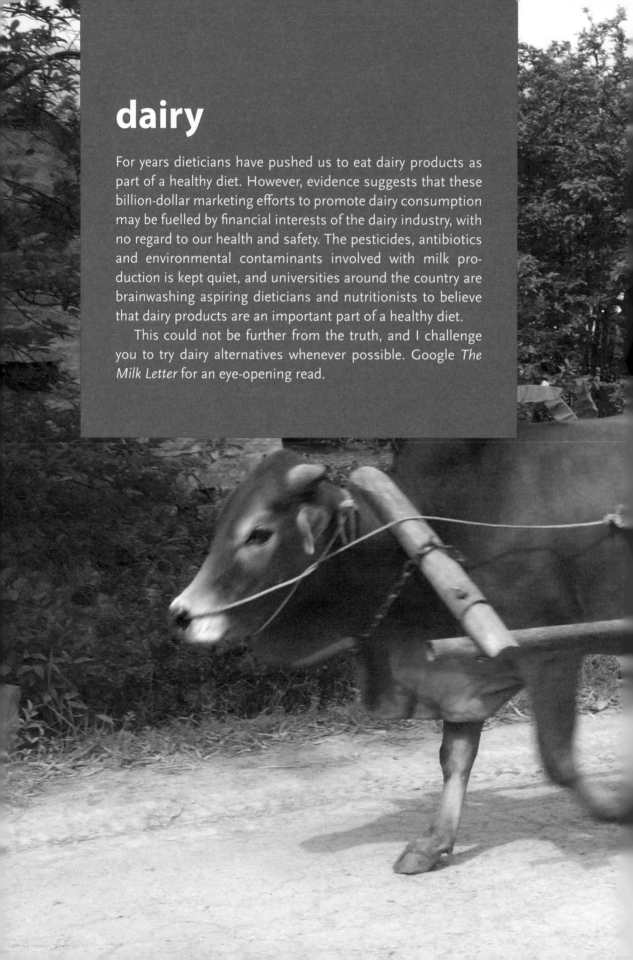

dairy

For years dieticians have pushed us to eat dairy products as part of a healthy diet. However, evidence suggests that these billion-dollar marketing efforts to promote dairy consumption may be fuelled by financial interests of the dairy industry, with no regard to our health and safety. The pesticides, antibiotics and environmental contaminants involved with milk production is kept quiet, and universities around the country are brainwashing aspiring dieticians and nutritionists to believe that dairy products are an important part of a healthy diet.

This could not be further from the truth, and I challenge you to try dairy alternatives whenever possible. Google *The Milk Letter* for an eye-opening read.

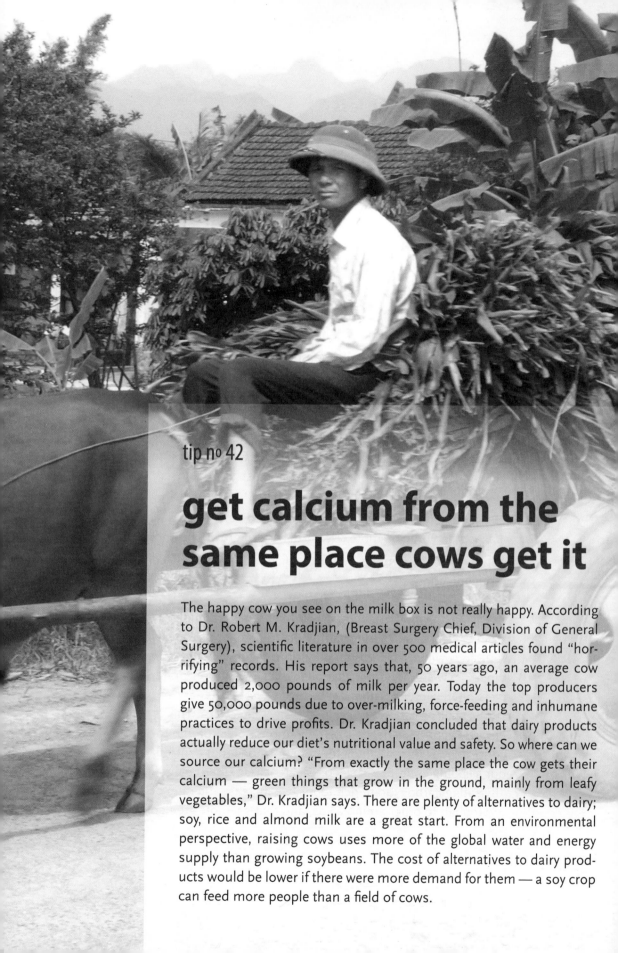

tip nº 42

get calcium from the same place cows get it

The happy cow you see on the milk box is not really happy. According to Dr. Robert M. Kradjian, (Breast Surgery Chief, Division of General Surgery), scientific literature in over 500 medical articles found "horrifying" records. His report says that, 50 years ago, an average cow produced 2,000 pounds of milk per year. Today the top producers give 50,000 pounds due to over-milking, force-feeding and inhumane practices to drive profits. Dr. Kradjian concluded that dairy products actually reduce our diet's nutritional value and safety. So where can we source our calcium? "From exactly the same place the cow gets their calcium — green things that grow in the ground, mainly from leafy vegetables," Dr. Kradjian says. There are plenty of alternatives to dairy; soy, rice and almond milk are a great start. From an environmental perspective, raising cows uses more of the global water and energy supply than growing soybeans. The cost of alternatives to dairy products would be lower if there were more demand for them — a soy crop can feed more people than a field of cows.

sleep more, weigh less

Catching a good night's sleep does more than make you feel rested and energized. Sleep is also a powerful regulator of appetite and weight control — studies have found the more that people lack sleep, the more likely they are to become overweight.

benefits of sleep

- Improved ability to learn new tasks and remember what you have learned. A lack of sleep can cause us to make decisions much slower; also these decisions tend to be faulty and can become more about risk taking.
- Reduced stress and health complications. A lack of sleep places the body under stress and may trigger the release of stress-related hormones that can cause unwarranted increases in both heart rate and blood pressure.
- Some studies have also shown that people who chronically lack sleep have higher blood levels of C-reactive protein. Higher levels of this protein may suggest a greater risk of developing hardening of the arteries (atherosclerosis).
- Better ability to repair muscles, damaged cells and tissues. Deep sleep triggers more release of human growth hormone.
- Strengthened immune system, which helps fight off common infections.

Including carb-rich foods in your diet (such as whole grains, rice, pasta, hummus and non-dairy milk) provides your body with the serotonin needed to regulate appetite and mood. New studies show that people on low-carbohydrate diets often wind up with a deficiency in serotonin that can start a chain reaction of interrupted sleeping cycles. This is because your body needs a certain amount of serotonin to convert efficiently into melatonin (a hormone that controls our sleeping cycle). Says sleep researcher Dr. Charli Sargent, "By eating carbohydrate-rich foods, we increase the ratio of tryptophan to other amino acids, and that promotes the entry of tryptophan into the brain, and then the next step is serotonin and promoting sleep."

Eating foods that contain tyramine earlier on in the day can help. Tyramine is an amino acid that causes the release of a brain stimulant, which makes you feel alert and keeps you up at night. Bananas, nuts, vanilla, figs, raisins, beer, wine, red pepper, tomatoes, soy sauce, red plums, eggplants and chocolate all contain tyramine.

tip n⁰ 43

low-fat dairy is better

If you choose to include dairy in your diet, choose lower-fat options. Use fresh fruit for flavor to minimize sugar content. Try different brands until you find your favorite, keeping fat count below 2%.

Although made from dairy, whipped cream, butter, sour cream and cream cheese are considered fat sources due to their high fat content, over-riding the good of the calcium and vitamin D. Treat dairy products as an occasional treat — source your calcium from green leafy vegetables and go outside for your vitamin D!

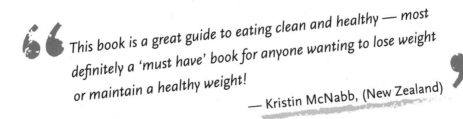

This book is a great guide to eating clean and healthy — most definitely a 'must have' book for anyone wanting to lose weight or maintain a healthy weight!

— Kristin McNabb, (New Zealand)

tip n⁰ 44

drink less milk

Choose options with lower lactose levels as this is a sugar that can cause bloating and discomfort. Choose a milk or milk alternative with less than 2 grams of fat and less than 100 calories per serving — many non-dairy milks have added sugar and flavorings. Watch the sugar, plain is best. Check out low-fat almond, coconut, rice and lactose-free varieties. Buy certified organic milk and dairy products. Organic animals can only be fed 100% organic feed and cannot be given antibiotics or growth hormones.

Some hormones that may be used in dairy cows include:

- Recombinant bovine growth hormone (rbGH) — to promote milk production (also known as bovine somato-tropin [BST]).
- Estrogen, testosterone and progesterine — steroid hormones added to promote growth and production.

Organic dairy farms do not allow the use of rBGH, and other companies that do not use rBGH often include this information on the label. It is also safe to buy imported European Union and Canadian cheeses and other dairy products, as rbGH is banned in these countries.

rBST has not been allowed on the market in Canada, Australia, New Zealand, Japan, Israel and all European Union countries. In the United States, the FDA stated that food products made from rBST-treated cows are "safe for human consumption, and no statistically significant differences exist between milk derived from rBST-treated and non-rBST-treated cows."

In response to concerns, some retailers now publish policies on use of rBST in production of milk products, while others try their hardest to assure the public that milk from rBST-treated cows is safe.

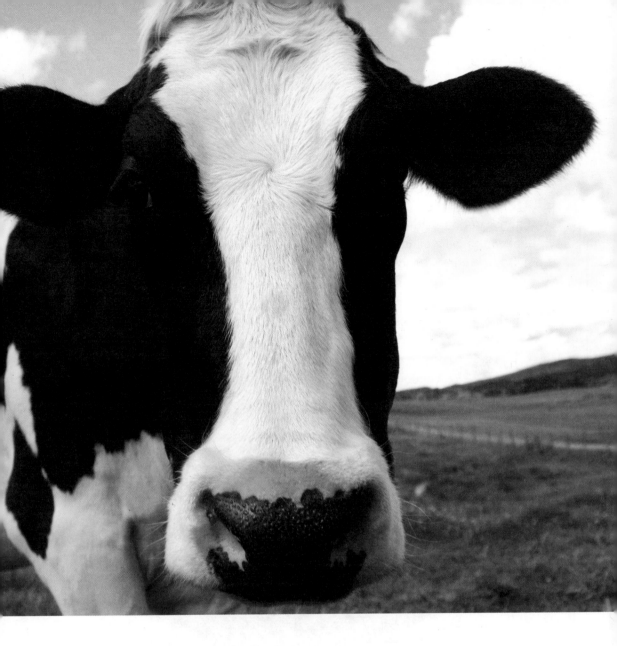

tip n⁰ 45

eat soft cheese

Calories vary according to the type of milk the cheeses are made from.
For the lowest fat content, choose the low-fat soft cheeses, cottage cheese
or yogurt cheese made from low-fat or skimmed milk. Lowest among the
semi-hard cheeses is camembert, and among the hard cheeses, edam or
gouda.

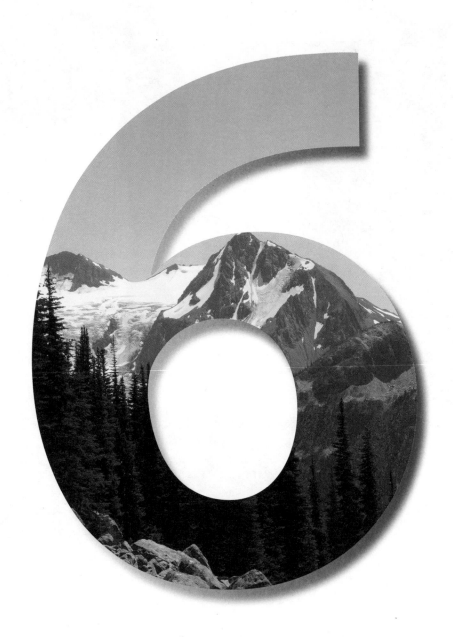

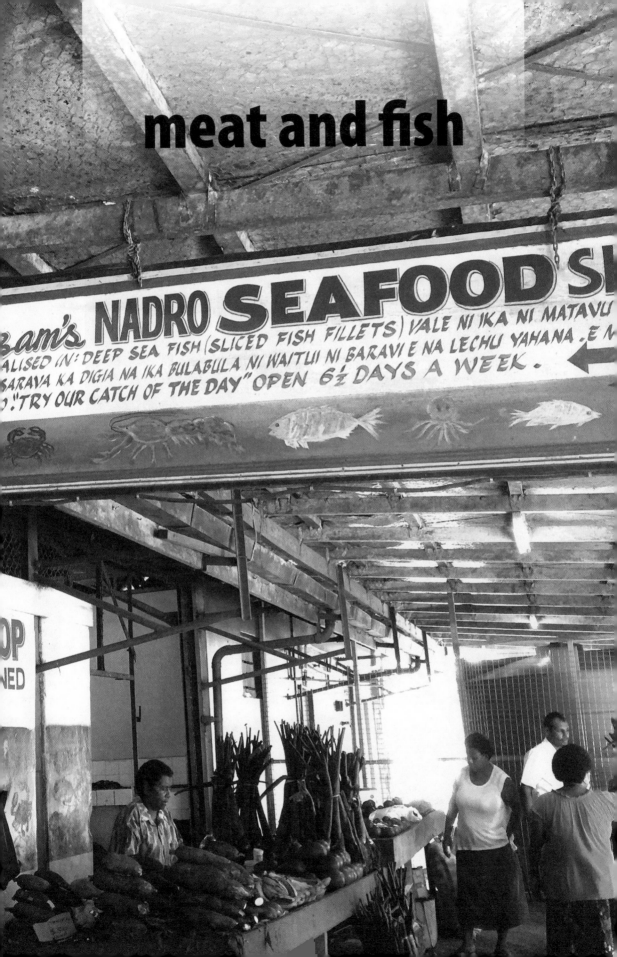

meat and fish

meat

Overconsumption of meat has become part of today's culture, and we are socially conditioned to eat it in most cases. *The Planet Friendly Diet* is about choosing eco-best fish and plant-protein-combining techniques to lose weight and save the world!

When meat is overemphasized in a person's diet, there are risks associated with increased protein and fats intake, especially red meat. According to one study of 62,582 men and women participants following a low-carbohydrate and high-protein diet, with a follow-up of 17.8 years, there is increased risk of general cancer and respiratory cancer. Often people who eat too much meat do not balance out their carbohydrates in healthy accordance with the macronutrient ratio outlined at the beginning of this book, which can increase production of C-reactive protein (causative agent of inflammation).

Going low-carb and high-protein might accelerate weight loss in the short term; however, it can increase the risk of cardiovascular conditions in the process. Vegetarian protein sources are usually rich in complex carbohydrates that provide the body with the balanced meal needed to function at optimal level.

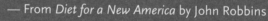

"When most of us sit down to eat, we aren't very aware of how our food choices affect the world. We don't realize that in every Big Mac there is a piece of the tropical rainforests, and with every billion burgers sold another hundred species become extinct. We don't hear the cry of the hungry millions who might otherwise be fed. But once we become aware of the impact of our food choices, we can never really forget."

— From *Diet for a New America* by John Robbins

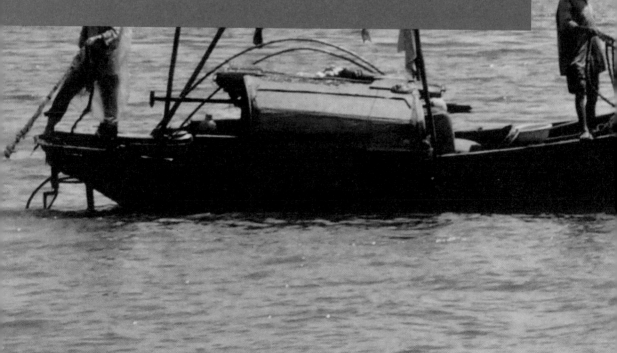

There is enough medical evidence to suggest that red meat should be avoided, even lean cuts.

Eating lean, grass-fed beef is a great start, but it's not a solution if you're eating too much of it. *The Planet Friendly Diet* will teach you loads of delicious ways to get your protein. Meat is only one way! And eating too much of it can contribute to health conditions like obesity, heart disease, cancer, diabetes, stroke, osteoporosis, hypertension, gallstones, kidney stones, hemorrhoids, high cholesterol, and depression. People usually wind up eating too much meat because everyone else is eating too much meat — it's part of our culture. But what's cool about that is we create our own culture! Meat eating is powered by appetite, not hunger. Your mind may crave it, but your body doesn't. Train your brain to stop thinking about it, and in a couple of weeks you'll hardly notice that you're not eating it. Just like cigarettes — it's a social conditioning.

> "Making meat-eating a social disgrace in this generation, just like we did with cigarette smoking in the last generation, is a fundamental change that must take place in order to advance our society to the next level and ensure our personal survival."
>
> — Dr John A. McDougall, M.D.

The global impact that meat eating has had on world hunger and the environment is endangering life as we know it. According to reports by the World Health Organization, overconsumption of meat is the major contributing factor to almost all categories of eco-disasters today. It's hands down the most "not green" thing you can do.

> "Earth provides enough to satisfy every man's need but not every man's greed."
>
> — Mahatma Gandhi

We can truly save the world, and we vote with our dollars. Choosing to buy meat is consequently choosing to tear down rainforests that thousands of animal species call home. You see, if there were less demand for meat production, there would be more land available for soybeans and other crops that provide sustainable protein sources for a vegetarian diet. Soybeans produce twice as much protein, per acre, than any other vegetable or grain crop, and about fifteen times more protein than land set aside for meat production. World hunger is unnecessary — there's enough to go around if we were all able to access our share.

So just like a bag of potato chips, if you are going to eat land animals, save them for a special occasion. Be conscious of your choices.

tip no 46

choose eco-best fish

Choose wild fish from healthy, well-managed populations caught using gear that does little harm to sea life and marine habitats. Or pick farmed fish raised in systems that control pollution, the spread of disease, chemical use and escaped fish. If it is farmed, it should be raised in a less harmful tank or pond. Avoid buying large slow-growing species as they are more vulnerable to overfishing. Good choices include wild Alaskan salmon, Pacific halibut, sole and long-line-caught Alaskan cod. These are firm fishes, good for cooking, as they hold their structure and don't shrink too much. Check out the list of eco-best choices at edf.org. Most fish on this list are low in environmental contaminants and can be safely eaten at least once per week. When buying ahi tuna (yellow-fin), ask your fishmonger for fish caught by trolling or pole-and-line gear (especially from the U.S. Atlantic), as their fishing practices result in almost no bycatch (no living creatures have been caught unintentionally by fishing gear, like dolphins in a trawling net). If this is not available locally, chose albacore.

> check out eco-best
> fish choices at edf.org.

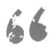 *I wanted to be prepared to work with Cat Smiley on my trip to Whistler Fitness Vacations to start my life style change so I ordered this book — it's easy to read with some delicious recipes! I read it from cover to cover in two days — I tried several recipes and they are delicious. I love the weekly shopping lists — it really helps with the planning. The Planet Friendly Diet is a great blueprint to help me along.*
— Sonya Olson, Florida (USA)

1 serving is enough

Learn your portion sizes and stick to them. Portions are usually driven by appetite, not hunger. Eat slowly, enjoy your meal and listen to your body. We really don't need too much food.

- 3 to 4 ounces of cooked fish, shellfish, poultry or lean meat

- ¾ cup of cooked legumes

- ½ package of tofu

- 2 eggs

- ¼ cup of shelled nuts

question big brother

There is evidence to suggest that the political power of food and agricultural associations often influences our government's food nutrition guidelines, which usually lean towards the industry that will help boost the nation's economy, not necessarily our health. For example, milk companies have been accused of influencing the *United States Department of Agriculture* into making the colored spots on the newly created food pyramid larger for their particular product. There is argument that the milk section is the easiest to see out of the 6 sections of the pyramid, making people believe that more milk should be consumed on a daily basis compared to other food groups. This also implies that the inclusion of milk is a necessary part of a healthy diet, which we've learned is simply not the case.

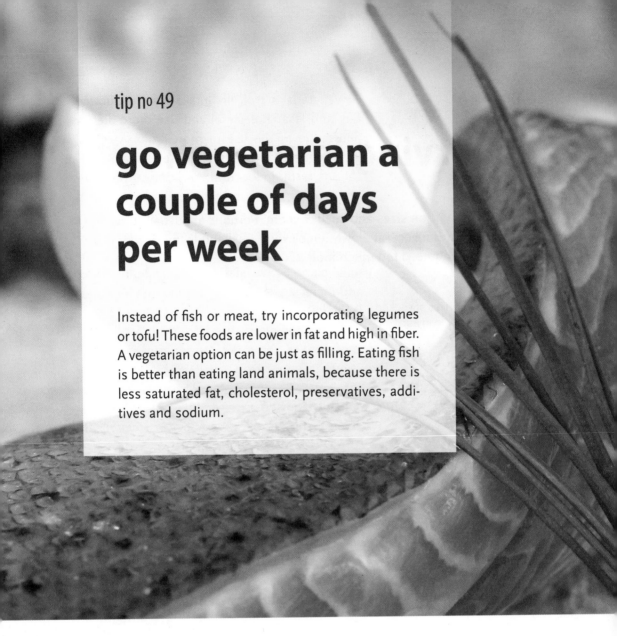

tip nº 49

go vegetarian a couple of days per week

Instead of fish or meat, try incorporating legumes or tofu! These foods are lower in fat and high in fiber. A vegetarian option can be just as filling. Eating fish is better than eating land animals, because there is less saturated fat, cholesterol, preservatives, additives and sodium.

Approximately 2.4% of adults in the United States and 4% adults in Canada are vegetarian. There are 3 classes:

lacto-ovo no fish and red meat. Protein sources include dairy products, beans, legumes, eggs, nuts and pulses.

lacto no eggs, fish and red meat. Protein sources include dairy products, legumes, beans, nuts and pulses.

vegan no animals or animal by-products. Protein sources include plant-based food only, namely nuts, beans, legumes, non-dairy milk and pulses.

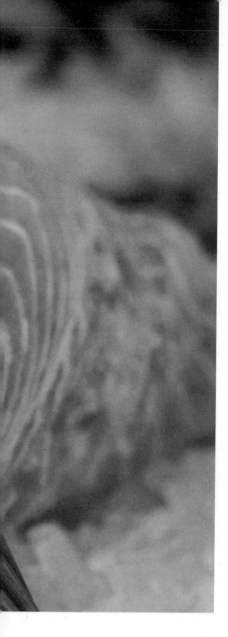

Vegetarians typically intake fewer saturated fats and less cholesterol and use more dietary fibers due to the use of more fruits, veggies, nuts, legumes and pulses. These eating modifications result in low BMI, lower blood pressure and low ischemic heart rate deaths and reduced incidence of diseases and conditions like hypertension, diabetes mellitus type 2, cancers and stroke compared to the meat eaters. With proper meal planning, vegetarians can lead a healthier and increasingly disease-free life, in addition to living longer.

Questions often arise from avid meat eaters and skeptics about the deficiency of protein in vegetarianism. This is usually because they know someone who perhaps "went vegetarian" without educating themselves in nutrition science, therefore not knowing how to balance their meals correctly or plan. As a result, they may have had health complications resulting from deficiencies in proteins, calcium, iron, zinc, vitamins A and B12. However, this won't happen to you because you're taking the time to read and learn how to do it properly with the lessons outlined in my fabulous book! Trust me, you're going to be okay. More than okay. You're going to feel amazing on both a physical and spiritual level because it really feels kinder to not contribute to animals being killed for our taste preferences. You'll learn to enjoy plant-based protein just as much as meat-based protein and probably wonder why you ever ate so much meat in the first place.

tip nº 50

trim visible fat

If you decide to go back to eating meat after your 21 days on *The Planet Friendly Diet*, choose leaner cuts that have little to no visible fat. Before cooking, trim all visible fat. Removing the fat after cooking is not recommended, as the fat has already leached into the meat.

Leaner cuts of meat are better, such as beef eye of round, skinless chicken breast, pork tenderloin, white turkey meat and wild salmon fillet. Choose the leanest ground beef possible — the extra money you spend will save your heart from gobs of saturated fat. Even better, instead of beef, try ground white chicken meat, turkey or even salmon. The variety in tastes will add twists to your old favourite recipes.

When preparing the meat, use healthful cooking methods that won't add unnecessary fat and calories. Try roasting or grilling the meat. This will let the excess fat drain off. Poaching salmon or chicken in a rich and flavorful chicken or vegetable broth imparts loads of flavor without a lot of added calories.

action steps

- Cut the visible fat from the steak before cooking it — that way the fat does not get into the meat.

- Use lemon wedges or spices to season meat, seafood and shellfish instead of butter, hollandaise and béarnaise sauces.

- Braising lean cuts of meat, which are often more inexpensive than their fatty counterparts, will render the meat tender and juicy.

- Slow cookers are also a great way to tenderize leaner cuts of meat.

- Swap the usual chicken or beef in your meal for heart-healthy salmon or figure-friendly legumes or tofu.

- Avoid deep-fried meats: dry ribs, chicken wings, chicken strips and crunchy chicken sandwiches.

- Greatly limit your consumption of bacon. It counts as a fat serving, and it's chock full of lard. Canadian bacon or ham is a healthier substitute.

- Choose burgers without mayonnaise, sugary barbeque sauces or fried onions. Load up on veggies, mustard and tomato. Have your burger with a small salad or non-creamy soup. Even better, switch the beef burger for a salmon or veggie burger.

tip no 51

don't eat
processed meat

Processed meat is pure junk, filled with fillers, binders and loads of chemicals that flavor, color and preserve. Plus they're crazy high in sodium and fat — the silent killers. Bologna, pepperoni and salami are loaded with pork, beef, preservatives, additives, sodium and saturated fat. They have no place in a sandwich.

Instead choose sliced roasted turkey meat, Bavarian ham or white chicken meat. Avoid or limit sausages and bacon — choose leaner alternatives such as baked ham or roasted turkey sausages. You will get the benefit of flavor, without the fat, sodium and excess calories.

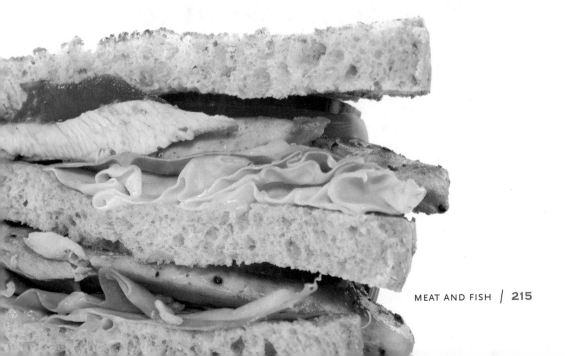

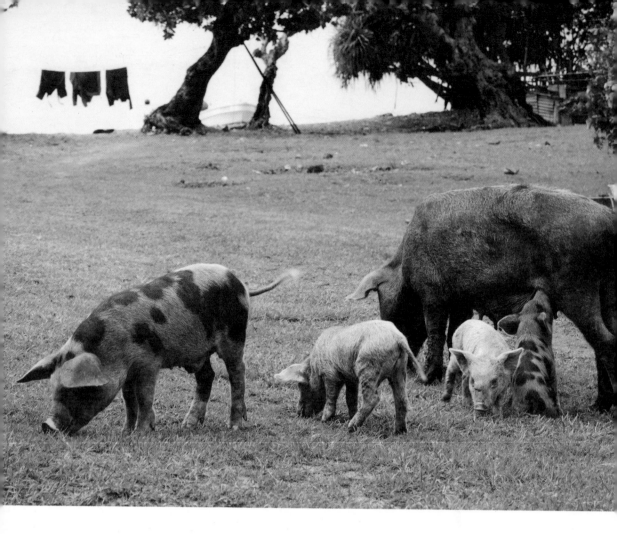

tip № 52

animals don't want to be eaten

If you're going to eat red meat, just eat it once in a while and make sure it comes from an animal that has been properly fed and raised (not on a factory farm).

living compassionately is about filling your plate with good karma food. If you're not concerned about the health benefits of eating less meat, spare a few thoughts for the planet and welfare of the creatures that share it with you.

tip nº 53

you are what you eat — do you want to be a cow?

When you eat meat, you are also ingesting herbicides, pesticides, synthetic fertilizers and the antibiotics and hormones given to animals to make them big and fat. Continued consumption of these animals will make you big and fat. Most studies on meat eating have not examined toxic chemical exposure.

As the human appetite for land animals increases, the production demand also increases, and farmers are using chemicals that were not known 40 years ago, which means that the long-term effects of exposure to these toxins may not yet be known. This is pretty risky!

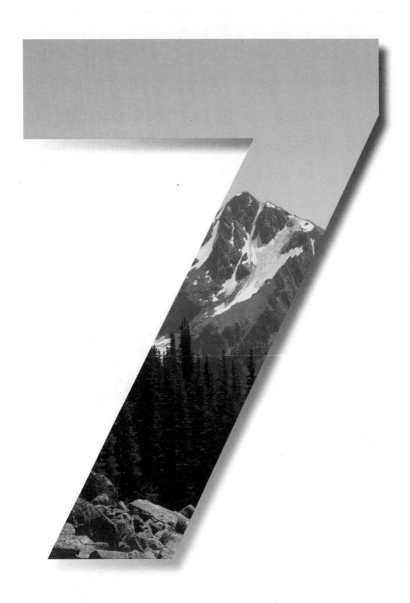

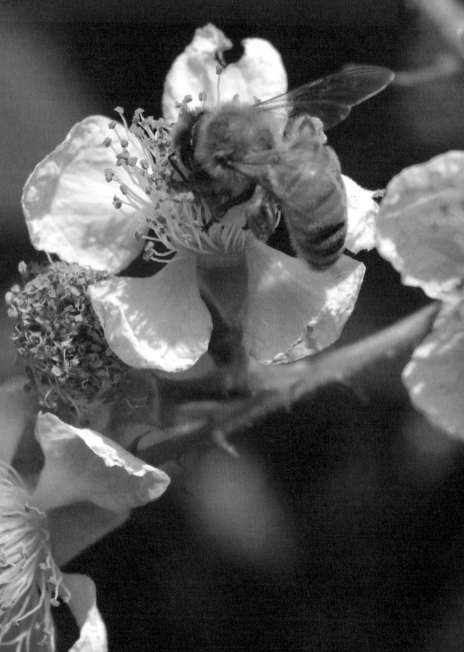

salt and sugar

salt

Salt is an important part of a healthy diet and can be found by eating balanced natural foods. Sodium helps regulate blood pressure and nerve fibers, as well as assisting cells in our body to function properly. The recommended intake is between 1,500 and 2,300 mg a day for healthy adults, according to the Canadian Hypertension Education Program. A 2004 Statistics Canada study found the average salt intake for Canadians was a whopping 3,092 mg — way more than the maximum recommended .

tip no 54

stay away from salt

It's recommended that we stick to less than 2,300 milligrams of sodium a day total. This includes the salt that is already in foods and any salt that you add at the dinner table. Even if you don't add it to your food, salt is everywhere... in everything that is not made from scratch in your kitchen.

Too much salt in your system causes extra water to stay in your body. This makes you thirstier as you are not getting the hydration that you need to make things run smoothly. It's not healthy to feel bloated after a meal or have swollen fingers. This water weight will naturally flush itself out in a few hours.

Although there are no calories in salt, cutting back will naturally decrease your body weight.

Imagine a river running through a tunnel — everything flows smoothly on a normal day. But when there is a storm, the river runs too high for the tunnel to support the raging torrent... and may collapse under pressure.

Your blood pressure is like that river, and the arteries are the tunnel. When you're healthy, your heart pumps blood into your arterial wall just fine. When you eat too much salt, your blood volume will increase due to excess water retention or because the blood vessels have constricted, putting pressure against the arterial walls. It's only understandable that eventually your arteries will freak out and get so damaged that a heart attack, stroke (brain attack) or kidney disease will be unavoidable.

Salt is the "silent killer" because you do not realize you have high blood pressure until you get your blood pressure reading or you have a heart attack. People usually don't realize that they are eating too much salt, and high blood pressure has no symptoms.

There are some factors that increase your likelihood of developing high blood pressure that cannot be controlled, such as age (older people are more likely to develop high blood pressure), race (African-Americans are at an increased risk) and heredity (high blood pressure runs in the family).

action steps

Factors that influence your blood pressure:

- Obesity: More than 60% of high blood pressure cases are in overweight people. Losing weight can significantly reduce blood pressure.
- Sodium consumption: Reducing salt intake can lower your blood pressure.
- Minerals: Consuming fruits and vegetables can often counteract the sodium that raises blood pressure.
- Smoking: In the short term, smoking can increase blood pressure.
- Oral contraceptives: Women who take birth control may develop high blood pressure.
- Physical inactivity: Lack of exercise can contribute to high blood pressure.

I'm really happy with The Planet Friendly Diet, I came to Whistler Fitness Vacations from Pakistan and have to say, I love all of the recipes — they were written very clearly. I loved the zero-waste principal of this diet, I was not vegetarian by any means before I started this plan, but it's made me really taste food again and above all, enjoy eating. I used to get headaches but now I don't get any headaches. I am really looking forward to guiding my family members on how to measure, eat proper portions and choose healthier ingredients based on what is important for their bodies. Whatever I have learnt while following this book I feel like I can pass it on to people back home. Thank you Cat!"

— Myrah Osman, Pakistan

tip № 55

get your blood pressure tested

You'll get two numbers: systolic and diastolic. The larger top number, the systolic pressure, represents the pressure that is in your arteries while your heart beats. The smaller bottom number, the diastolic pressure, is the number to really be concerned with. It is the pressure while your heart is relaxing between beats. A normal blood pressure reading for an adult should be below 140/90.

> these days, you can check your blood pressure at most drug stores and pharmacies — or ask your doctor if you're in the healthy zone.

 check out these sodium counts!

- 3 oz salami: 1,922 mg

- 1 cup chicken noodle soup: 1,106 mg

- 1 teaspoon regular soy sauce: 1,029 mg

- 1 oz pretzels: 476 mg

- 30 g Special K cereal: 306 mg

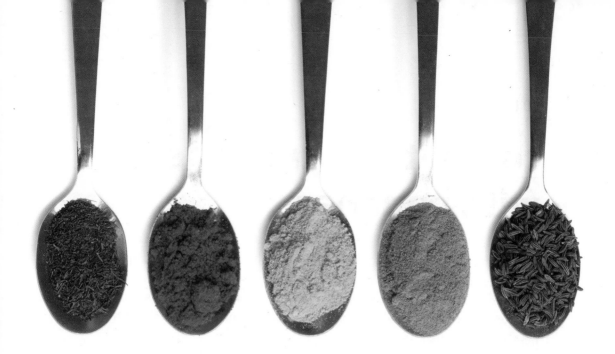

tip №56

packaged foods are not worth their salt

The average North American gets 75% of their daily salt intake from eating processed convenience foods in the form of prepackaged meals, canned soups, crackers, pasta sauces, chips, pretzels, frozen dinners, pickles and other food-like substances. This salt is added by manufacturers because they know that people love the taste of salt.

About 15% of our intake is added at the table from the salt shaker. The remaining 10% is from natural unprocessed foods that are also high in the counteracting mineral, potassium.

action step

Limit processed, packaged foods — read the nutrition label and look for the lowest sodium option.

Try dried herbs and spices, garlic, vinegar and lemons in place of salt. Eat more unprocessed whole foods like fruit, vegetables and grain products.

tip nº 57

combat salt cravings with bananas

Combating salt cravings is not just about willpower — understanding what triggers the desire to overeat will help you stop it. Simply put, if you are eating too much salt, the body tries to get rid of the excess by sweating it out. Sweating is nature's way to get rid of the mineral electrolytes that help your body distribute fluids.

As with any food addiction, the body becomes reliant on salt to maintain a balance if it has become used to excess, so there will be some side effects when you withdraw. Increase potassium levels to combat these symptoms; shakes with banana, blue-green algae, yogurt and protein can help cut the cravings for high-salt foods — as can fish, olives, tomatoes, seaweed-based products and celery.

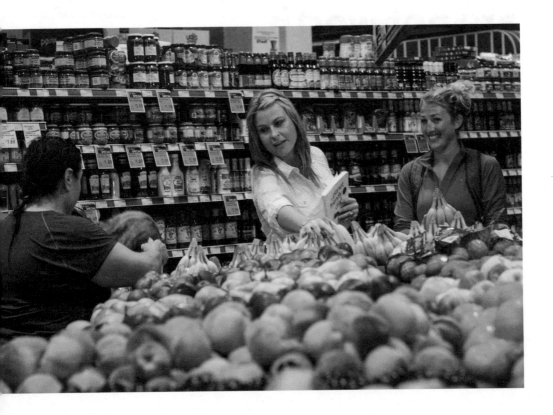

sugar

The whole food revolution has bought us healthier alternatives to chemically tampered sweeteners, allowing us to eat less, as they are naturally sweeter.

Unrefined sugars always have the country of origin and the name of the packer. They won't have a list of ingredients, because there aren't any.

Honey is your best natural sweetener as it is packed with vitamins and goodness. Honey, like raw sugar, is high in calories but has its place in a healthy diet when used in moderation.

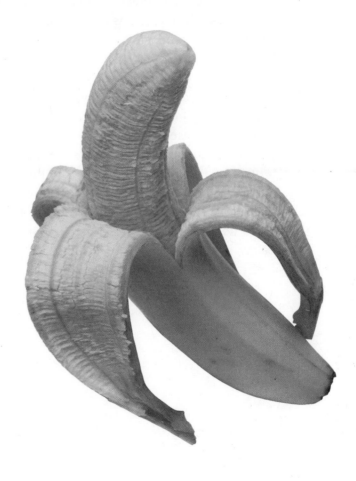

tip no 58

the more sugar you eat, the more you'll want to eat

Unfortunately, most of the best-tasting foods out there have some combination of sugar, fat or salt... the melt-in-your-mouth moment that arouses your senses when you have that first bite of chocolate cake stimulates the appetite and desire for more.

The combination of sugar and fat is the most palatable taste, and sugar addiction is tough to break because of it; so you need to go into recovery with the same headspace as a cigarette smoker trying to quit.

Despite what people say, food addictions are not about willpower. Humans are emotional beings, with associated memories of high-fat, high-sugar foods. Our bliss point is one bite into a piece of dairy milk chocolate. Home sweet home! So if you're really serious about losing weight and recovering from sugar addiction, stop being face-to-face with it. Do not go on a cruise ship. Avoid all-inclusive vacations. Quit your waitress job. Dump your boyfriend who doesn't support your health goals.

Just like alcoholics who can't go to the bar, food addicts can't say no to fat and sugar combinations that are free and available once they have a lifetime of memories. There is no "everything in moderation" if you are a food addict, until you've retrained your brain and behavior to have a healthy relationship with food. Don't try to overcome food addictions alone — get professional help.

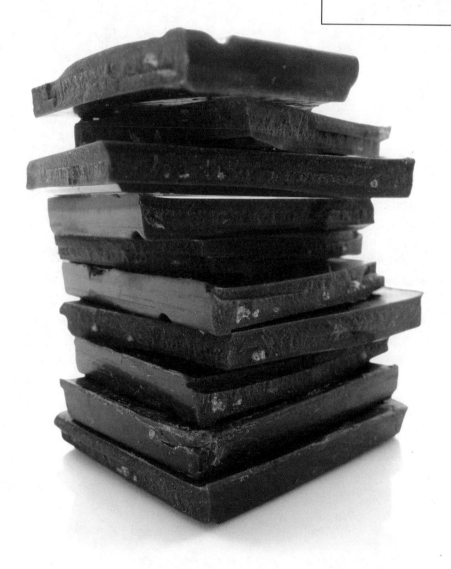

if you're really serious about losing weight and recovering from sugar addiction, stop being face-to-face with it.

tip nº 59

herbs and spices are better than ketchup

Try these natural seasoning options for a healthy low-fat kick to your dishes.

curries are popular dishes that can get pretty high in calories if you mix the traditional way with full-fat coconut milk. Use low-fat curry paste and mix it with non-dairy milk. Adding a spoonful of shredded coconut is an easy light way to stay low-fat without compromising flavor. You can also use curry powder, but most beginners find low-fat curry paste the easiest way to start.

jalapeño pepper has thermogenic properties that increase your fat-burning ability and metabolism. It's hot and spicy, but that's why we love it. Build your tolerance up gradually! The red peppers that you'll use in the salsa tend to be sweet — choose brightly colored peppers and store unwrapped in the fridge.

paprika spice is made from ground chili peppers — a sweeter, milder version of the jalapeño pepper. It is high in vitamin C and great used with hotter spices, like cayenne pepper. Taste a little bit on your tongue first before adding to the pan. Even people that don't like their food very spicy enjoy the kick from a pinch of paprika. Many get addicted!

turmeric is one of the most powerful spices, best known for its anti-inflammatory properties. The Chinese use it to treat depression. It is an earthy, gingery taste — almost bitter —

with a definite medicinal aftertaste if you use too much. Start with half a teaspoon.

chili spice is much hotter than paprika. It is definitely an acquired taste but, like paprika, is bursting with nutritional benefits. Your metabolism is boosted for about twenty minutes after eating spicy food — the body is burning calories to produce heat! Use in low dosages to start.

cumin is a pungent curry spice available as a ground powder or dried seed. It goes great with fresh cilantro and is best lightly roasted. Cumin is renowned as a powerful digestive aid, often regarded as a cleansing spice for its diuretic properties.

cilantro (coriander) is a great way to cool down hot spices! It goes perfectly with jalapeño and paprika. Daily use promotes clear radiant skin and reduced risk of skin cancer due to its ability to trap the free radicals caused by exposure to the sun. It also helps weight loss as it has been known to reduce the body's absorption of saturated fat.

tip nº 60

keep sugar to 10% of your daily total

Many processed foods have the dietary balance upside down. They give us instant energy in the form of concentrated sugar — wasted calories — and yet starve us of the natural nutrients and dietary fiber we need.

Perfect eating is not the goal, and it's unrealistic to strive for that. Instead, aim to keep a maximum of 10% of your daily calorie total for sugar-based treats. For example, if you're on a 1,200-calorie diet, keep sugar to 120 calories. Savour treats as treats by saving them for special occasions. Everything else you eat should be healthy and wholesome.

There is no such thing as a "bad" food, as everything can be enjoyed in moderation, as long as you are able to keep it in moderation.

perfect eating is not the goal, and it's unrealistic to strive for that.

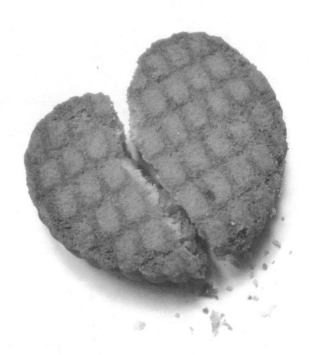

tip nº 61

know when to ride out your cravings... and when to give in

Set boundaries. If you want chocolate, eat a small piece. If you want more, have a glass of water and get away from the food. You'll enjoy the taste more when you're able to savour it.

Listen to your body. If your stomach is rumbling before you go to bed, eat! Choose serotonin-rich foods with higher carbohydrate, such as cereal with non-dairy milk. The next day, you'll likely not be very hungry, but eat anyway. Skipping meals causes your blood sugar levels to plunge, making you likely to overeat later. Eat a little less and gear yourself up to get back on track.

Avoid after-dinner cravings by arming yourself with distraction tools — the worst thing you can do is sit on the sofa and watch TV. Marketing experts know when we're at our most vulnerable! Instead make yourself a pot of herbal tea or brush your teeth. Gain closure on your eating for the day with something minty — it doesn't go so well with food. Clean the kitchen and put away leftovers so you won't be tempted to pick. Take the dog out for a long walk or call a friend. If you want to keep dessert as part of your ritual, have a piece of fruit or a scoop of sorbet.

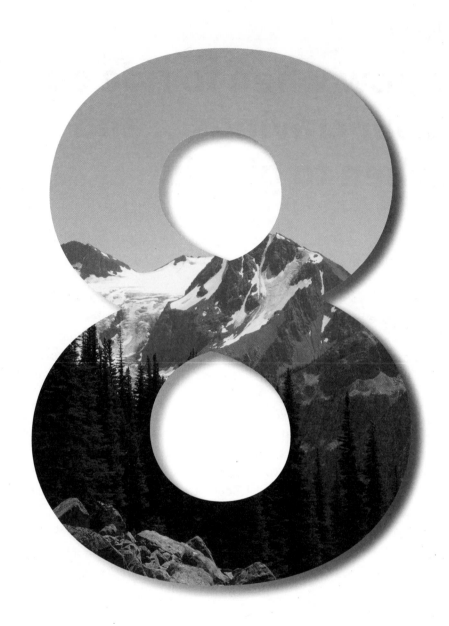

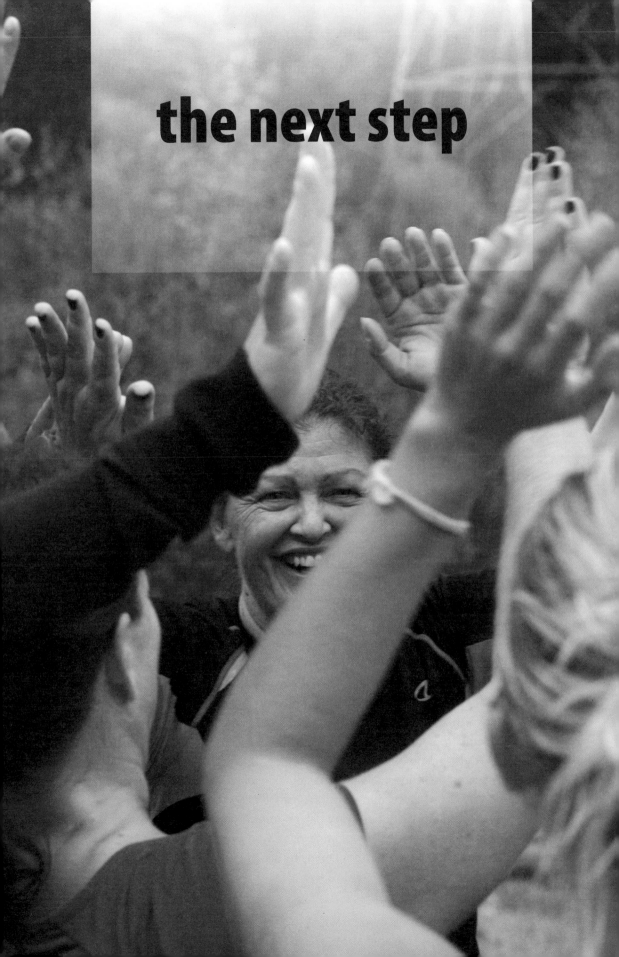

the next step

tip nº 62

make it your own

Over the years, I've coached hundreds of beautiful women to slim down to their happy size, and stay there. They were just like me: rebels at heart, with no intention of following someone else's "rules." The last thing I want to do is tell people what to do. You want to eat whatever the heck you want...right? Right!

The recipes in this book are intended as an example of how to make your own meals, for the rest of your life. It's only intended to be followed once, or for as long as you're at *Whistler Fitness Vacations*. From there, you make your own recipes! Just make sure you've memorized the three fundamental principles (page 130) and that you apply them to every meal. *The Planet Friendly Diet* is an awesome collection of recipes with a fusion of international flavors and modern taste that you can apply it to your own culture, traditions, tastes and preferences. Empowered eating is about taking charge of your food choices — having the strength and courage to try new things and make changes. Embrace the challenge like a new chapter in your life, taking time to put fresh wholesome foods together.

Guests at my weight-loss retreat usually continue on this way of "almost vegetarian" eating plan periodically, while others reintroduce gluten, wheat, dairy and animals into their diet. Whatever you decide, we recommend that you make any changes slowly, as sugar, fat, salt and other foods that you haven't been eating while on this plan may cause your body to reject them to some degree.

This book is a road map towards finding time for yourself, learning to cook, loving your body, being greener, trying new adventures, getting fit, losing weight, eating better, saving money, taking risks and following a journey that matches your core values.

Much care has been taken to plan each dish so that it is rich in antioxidants, vitamins and minerals, with limited saturated fat; more fruit, vegetables, legumes, nuts, grains, heart-healthy oils and fish. It's a little bit of a beauty boot camp too; hair and nails grow faster, skin will glow while you feast on super-foods. We don't encourage puritanical behavior, but encourage people to spend 10% of their calories every day on lovable foods, such as a slice of cheese, some chocolate, glass of wine or maybe even a burger or chicken wings on occasion. We are all about enjoying life, and food is a big part of that.

Daily nutritional goals:

- 4 liters of water (1 liter during your workout).
- Wake up in the morning hungry and ready for breakfast.
- Eat 2 meals with cutlery.
- Drink fewer than 6 alcoholic beverages each week.
- Take 20 minutes to eat each meal.

Our goal at *Whistler Fitness Vacations* is to reset your metabolism, so if you go back to regular meat eating, we recommend you keep the portions under 4 ounces. Select grass-fed organic meats with the lowest fat content; discard all the visible fat, and make grilling your first option when eating red and smoked meats to avoid hidden fats.

There's a lot of hype out there at the moment about why it's better to eat less meat. This book is not intended to convince you to go vegetarian, it's meant as kind of a "catchall" net of those who have already been exposed to all the nasty facts through channels such as TED talks, documentaries, social media etc. Most people find that after a couple of weeks on *The Planet Friendly Diet* they think twice about how much meat they are eating, opting for more plant-based options when they can. Chicken could replace white fish, beef could replace salmon, and egg whites could replace tofu. Keep consumption to a minimum, with one meat meal (tops) per day. Try Monday, Wednesday and Friday having fish dinners, Tuesday and Thursday having chicken dinners, Saturday having red meat (burger, etc.), and on Sunday going vegan.

Continue the smoothies for as long as you like; it's an amazing way to eat well when on the go. Stay on 1,200 calories until you reach goal weight, to a maximum of 60 days, and then increase the portions for a more moderate-paced weight loss. You can also switch out just one meal per day for a smoothie, for example, having regular meals for lunch and dinner and a smoothie for breakfast.

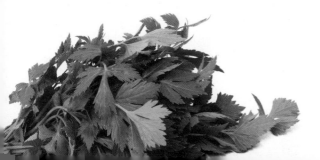

tip n⁰ 63

wake up. kick-ass — repeat (for life)

Over the few weeks on *The Planet Friendly Diet,* your body will have started rebuilding its cell structure and forming new habits. If you're now going off the plan, be sure to check the page just before this one for some tips on how to maintain your current weight. If you simply stop training, then your body will progressively gain weight because you will not have the same calorie burn and your metabolism won't reach the same peaks as it would if you were exercising.

It's important to eat smart and exercise at least one hour per day, five days per week, to continue on your weight-loss journey or maintain your optimal weight. Our goal is for you to make this a way of life. The secret to achieving your goals is mapping out a realistic plan to attainment, with measured success. Be specific — break it down to weekly goals, like running 3 times a week for 30 minutes or walking the dog every day for an hour before work.

Most guests at *Whistler Fitness Vacations* strive to slim down to their "happy weight" which is determined usually by 100 lb. for the first 5 feet, then 7 or 8 lb. per inch over, depending on their muscle mass and body structure. For example, a muscular woman of 5'5" would find her happy weight to be about 140 lb., which is what she should aim to stay at for life. If there is an event coming up, she would slim down to her "supermodel weight," which is 5 lb. lighter (135 lb.) by jumping on *The Planet Friendly Diet* again and aiming to stay at 135 lb. for no longer than 3 months. Her "scary weight" is 5 lb. heavier than her "happy weight" so if her weight gets up to 145 lb., she'd also get back onto the plan until she stabilizes again at her "happy weight."

Commit to putting into action the nutrition lessons that I've explained to you in this book; they really will help you come a long way in letting go of restrictive eating habits. The best thing is to listen to what your body really needs, and try to free yourself from the diet mentality. Be social — let me know how you are getting on. I'm here for you!

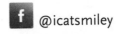 @icatsmiley

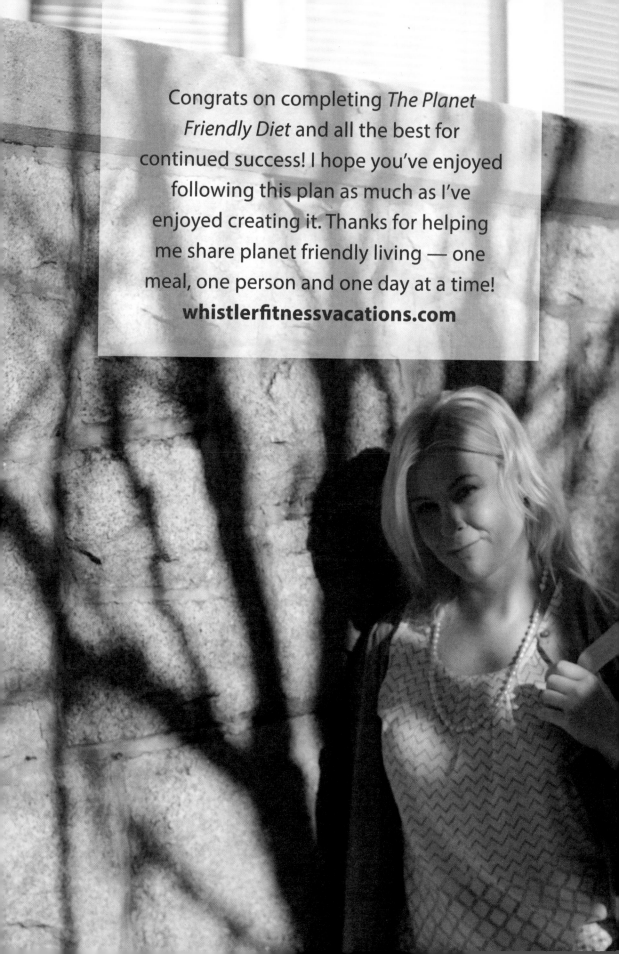

Congrats on completing *The Planet Friendly Diet* and all the best for continued success! I hope you've enjoyed following this plan as much as I've enjoyed creating it. Thanks for helping me share planet friendly living — one meal, one person and one day at a time!

whistlerfitnessvacations.com

index

potassium, 152, 155, 159, 167, 170, 175, 176, 223, 224
potatoes, 175
  neesuaz tuna salad, 80
  seared tuna harvest, 104
  simple salmon, 72
prepackaged meals, 223
probiotics, 177
processed foods, 177, 188, 215, 223, 230
protein powder, 25, 176.
  See also smoothies.
protein sources, 142, 208.
  See also black beans; eggs; legumes; meat; soybeans.
pulses, 138, 141, 184, 212

quesadilla, 30
quinoa, 1, 15–16, 27, 40, 56, 108, 112, 134, 143, 176, 188, 192
  edamame energizer, 64
  wonder bean quinoa, 76

recombinant bovine growth hormone (rbGH), 204
red cabbage, 176
  edamame energizer, 64
  sesame stir-fry, 88
red meat. *See* beef.
red onion, in salsa, 22
refined grains, 183, 186
refrigerating food, 10–11, 22, 23, 24, 56, 64, 168, 170, 171, 174, 176
riboflavin, 93, 184
rice, 23, 190. *See also* brown rice; curries.

salad dressing, 143, 165
salads
  baked salmon with spinach salad, 52
  neesuaz tuna salad, 80
salmon
  baked salmon with spinach salad, 52

remixed risotto, 112
  simple salmon, 72
  sock it to me salmon, 108
salsa, 21, 56, 137
  recipe, 22
salt, 170, 220–24. *See also* sodium.
Sargent, Charli, 202–03
saturated fats, 145, 146, 147, 155, 170, 177, 212, 213, 214, 215
seasonings, 223, 228–29
seitan, 52
serotonin, 93, 135, 136, 164, 202–03, 231
sesame seeds, 143, 146, 176
  sesame stir-fry, 88
shopping local, 8, 16, 164–65, 210
simple carbohydrates, 130, 134, 137
skin care, 14
sleep, 15, 93, 132, 133, 135, 136, 137, 202–03
smoking, 167, 221
smoothies, 7, 26, 27, 235
  alternative recipes, 28
  super smoothies, 25, 27, 144
snacks, 16, 21, 29, 33, 95, 130–31, 166, 170, 171, 174, 176
snap peas, 176
  baked salmon with spinach salad, 52
  festive tofu curry, 44
  sesame stir-fry, 88
sodas. *See* diet soft drinks.
sodium, 152, 159, 170, 185, 215, 220–21,
soluble fiber, 137, 195
soybeans, 177, 201, 209.
  See also edamame.
soy cheese, in neesuaz tuna salad, 80
soy foods, 177, 194
soy milk, 177, 194
spinach, 30, 35, 36, 152, 156, 163, 178, 198. *See also* green leafy vegetables.
  ahi steak with spicy rice, 40

bibliography

Adams, Jefferson. "Non-celiacs Benefit from Gluten-free Diet." *Celiacs Disease & Gluten Intolerance Research*. April 2009. Retrieved July 2010. www.celiacs.com/articles

Compassion in World Farming Trust. "Reducing Meat Consumption: The Case for Urgent Reform." 2004. Retrieved July 2010. www.ciwf.com

Dean, Amy and Jennifer Armstrong. "Genetically Modified Foods." *American Academy of Environmental Medicine*. May 2009. Retrieved July 2010. www.aaemonline.org

Department for Health and Human Services: Centers for Disease Control and Prevention. July 08, 2007. www.cdc.gov.

Eat Smart BC. "Eat Healthy, Be Safe." August 2010. Retrieved November 2010. www.eatsmartbc.ca

Fair Trade Network. "Where to Buy Fair Trade." 2010. Retrieved July 2010. www.fairtradesource.ca

Food and Agriculture Organization of the United Nation. Agriculture and Consumer Protection Department. "Livestock Impacts on the Environment." November 2006. Retrieved July 2010. www.fao.org

Greenpeace Canada. "How to Avoid Genetically Engineered Food: A Shopper's Guide." Retrieved July 2010. http://gmoguide.greenpeace.ca.

Health Canada. "Eating Well with Canada's Food Guide." www.hc-sc.gc.ca/fn-an/food-guide-aliment/index-eng.php. July 08, 2007.

Health Canada. "Whole Grains: Get the Facts." http://www.hc-sc.gc.ca/fn-an/nutrition/whole-grain-entiers-eng.php

Institute for Responsible Technology and the Non-GMO Project. "Non-GMO Shopping Guide." 2010. Retrieved July 2010. http://nongmosoppingguide.com

Korn, Danna. "Should You Be Wheat-free/Gluten-free?" Center for Celiac Research, Baltimore, MD. 2010. Retrieved July 2010. www.glutenfreedom.net

Kradjian, Robert M. "The Milk Letter: A Message to My Patients." 1995.

Mayo Clinic. "Mediterranean Diet: Ingredients for a Heart-Healthy Eating Approach." February 2010. Retrieved July 2010. www.mayoclinic.org

Mayo Clinic. "Meat-free More Often: Alternate Protein Sources Promote Health." May 2010. Retrieved July 2010. www.mayoclinic.org

McDougall, John A. "When Friends Ask: 'Why Did You Quit Meat?'" McDougall Newsletter. May 2007. Retrieved July 2010. www.drmcdougall.com

Pazderka, Catherine, Ann Rowan and Eric Enno Tamm. "The Green Guide to David Suzuki's Nature Challenge." 2003. Retrieved July 2010. http://www.davidsuzuki.org/publications/downloads/2003/GreenGuide.pdf

Pesticide Action Network North America. "What's on My Food? Wheat Flour: 16 Pesticides Found by United States Department of Agriculture Pesticide Data Program." 2010. Retrieved July 2010. www.whatsonmyfood.org

Robbins, John. *Diet for a New America: How Your Food Choices Affect Your Health, Happiness and the Future of Life on Earth,* 2nd Edition. Random House, 2006.

Schwartz, Rosie. "A Whole Grain of Truth." Retrieved May 1, 2007.

Sierra Club. "A True Picture of Meat and Dairy Consumption." Dallas-Fort Worth Earth. October 2010. Retrieved November 2010. www.dfwnetmall.com

Srivastava, K.C. and T. Mustafa. "Ginger (Zingiber officinale) in Rheumatism and Musculoskeletal Disorders," *Med Hypothesis*, 1992, 39, 342–348.

Starky, Sheena. "The Obesity Epidemic in Canada." Statistics Canada. July 2005. Retrieved July 2010. www2.parl.gc.ca

Suzuki, David. "More Vegetarians Needed." David Suzuki Foundation. October 2010. Retrieved November 2010. www.davidsuzuki.org/blogs

Usana Health Sciences. "Glycemic Index: From Research to Nutrition Recommendations?" Retrieved July 7, 2007.

U.S. Department of Agriculture. "Choose My Plate." Retrieved June 10, 2013. www.choosemyplate.gov/food-groups/grains-why.html.

U.S. Environmental Defense Fund. "How to Buy and Cook Seafood." January 1998. Retrieved July 2010. www.edf.org

U.S. Environmental Defense Fund. "Seafood Selector." November 2010. Retrieved November 2010. www.edf.org

Wigler I., I. Grotto, D. Caspi and M. Yaron. "The Effects of Zintona EC (a Ginger Extract) on Symptomatic Gonarthritis." *Osteoarthritis Cartilage*, November 2003, 11(11), 783–789.

"Whole Grain Foods and Heart Disease Risk." Retrieved March 29, 2009. www.ncbi.nlm.nih.gov/pubmed/10875600.

"Whole Grain Intake Is Favorably Associated with Metabolic Risk Factors for Type 2 Diabetes and Cardiovascular Disease in the Framingham Offspring Study." Retrieved February 30, 2009. www.ncbi.nlm.nih.gov/pubmed/12145012

Whole Grains Council. "Identifying Whole Grain Products." Retrieved February 2, 2008.

Whole Grains Council. "Intro to Whole Grains." Retrieved October 10, 2007.

Wood, Rebecca. *The Whole Foods Encyclopedia.* New York: Prentice-Hall, 1988.

World Health Organization. "Global Strategy on Diet, Physical Activity and Health." May 2004. Retrieved July 2010. www.who.intg

World Health Organization. "Obesity and Overweight." September 2006. Retrieved July 2010. www.who.int

World Health Organization. "10 Facts About Water Scarcity." March 2009. Retrieved July 2010. www.who.int

about the author

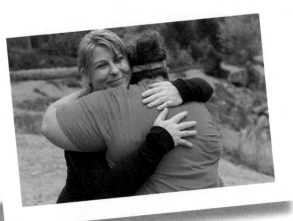

Cat Smiley is an award-winning personal trainer, weight-loss coach, health blogger and entrepreneur living in British Columbia. She has been named Canada's top trainer three times by the *International Sports Science Association (ISSA)*, recognized most for her work pioneering the nation's first fitness boot camp, The Original Boot Camp, in 2001. Her training methods focus on motivating, empowering and educating women to kick-start their change with simple lifestyle choices, building confidence and self-esteem.

Passionate about skiing, Cat grew up in the farmlands of New Zealand using back-to-basics workouts to achieve international heights in her athletic career. She was a professional skier and national team athlete for 12 years (achieving top 5 results in half-pipe World Cup, Global X Games, World Ski Invitational and US Open), enduring many long months of injury recoveries, including 22 broken bones and 3 knee operations. Following her debilitating head injury (that forced retirement months before the 1998 Olympics), doctors said that it "may be life-threatening to ski beyond an intermediate level again." They recommended rehabilitating her brain function through studying, which was a silver lining, as she took a break from sport to enroll in nutrition classes at Massey University...little did she know at the time that it would form the foundation for years to come!

She made an incredible comeback to professional skiing in 2001, moving from mogul skiing into "big mountain" competing, while launching her fitness trainer career in Canada. Her incredible story of determination, courage and tenacity landed her a starring role in the LIFE network reality show *Whistler Stories*, which was aired across North America in 2004.

Cat became well-known in her community and among friends for "moving bricks" — always questioning why the answer was "no" and working hard to find a way, no matter what. During her time as an athlete, she acquired valuable mental skills that she incorporates daily into her coaching techniques to inspire women to achieve their best, regardless of their physical restrictions and starting points. She quickly became a sought-after educator in the fitness industry, and co-authored the continuing certification course for boot camp instructors of the ISSA (an organization of almost 200,000 personal trainers in 28 countries), also publishing a book and DVD series on boot camp workouts. She ditched the camouflage and drill sergeant branding in 2012, packaging all services into her all-inclusive weight-loss retreat, *Whistler Fitness Vacations*. In the same year, she was recognized in the top 10 Boot Camp Instructors worldwide by IDEA trade publication, and approved by the USA and Canadian trademarks office to use the controversial **kick-ass workouts** as her authentic workout description.

These days, Cat Smiley is a certified Master Trainer (ISSA), developing and researching new programming ideas almost daily in fitness and nutrition, which she blogs on catsmiley.com. Her syndicated health columns have been featured in hundreds of Canadian community newspapers, and she frequently contributes to acclaimed publications including *Elle, Chatelaine, Canadian Living, Oxygen Magazine, SELF, Eat This Not That* and *Readers Digest.*

Whistler Fitness Vacations is Cat Smiley's fitness company; a residential weight-loss program with personal development coaching for improved health and lifestyle management. The program is designed to help women lead happier and healthier lives by getting them into top shape, regardless of their starting point. WFV is an accredited member of the Better Business Bureau with an A+ rating: fully insured, registered with the Province of British Columbia, and active members of the Chamber of Commerce as a licensed business in the Resort Municipality of Whistler (since 2001).

whistlerfitnessvacations.com

If you have enjoyed *The Planet Friendly Diet*, you might also enjoy other

BOOKS TO BUILD A NEW SOCIETY

Our books provide positive solutions for people who want to
make a difference. We specialize in:

**Food & Gardening • Resilience • Sustainable Building
Climate Change • Energy • Health & Wellness • Sustainable Living
Environment & Economy • Progressive Leadership • Community
Educational & Parenting Resources**

New Society Publishers

ENVIRONMENTAL BENEFITS STATEMENT

New Society Publishers has chosen to produce this book on recycled paper made with
100% post consumer waste, processed chlorine free, and old growth free.

For every 5,000 books printed, New Society saves the following resources:[1]

34	Trees
3,121	Pounds of Solid Waste
3,434	Gallons of Water
4,479	Kilowatt Hours of Electricity
5,673	Pounds of Greenhouse Gases
24	Pounds of HAPs, VOCs, and AOX Combined
9	Cubic Yards of Landfill Space

[1]Environmental benefits are calculated based on research done by the Environmental Defense Fund and
other members of the Paper Task Force who study the environmental impacts of the paper industry.

For a full list of NSP's titles, please call 1-800-567-6772 *or check out our website* at:

www.newsociety.com

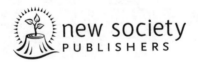

new society
PUBLISHERS